Heaven Touches Earth
Through Hospital Ministry

"I was sick and you visited me…"
Matthew 25:36

Heaven Touches Earth
Through Hospital Ministry

Handbook for Clergy and Lay Visitors

Derry James-Tannariello, MDiv., BCC

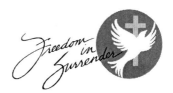

Mill City Press, Inc.
212 3rd Avenue North, Suite 290
Minneapolis, MN 55401
612.455.2294
www.millcitypublishing.com

Most scripture quotations are from *New King James Version* (NKJV) 1982 by Thomas Nelson, Inc., unless otherwise noted.

Some of the anecdotal illustrations in this book are true to life and are included with the permission of the persons involved. All other illustrations are composites of real situations, and any resemblance to people living or dead is coincidental.

For information regarding quantity discounts for bulk purchases for sales promotions, fund-raising, and educational needs, contact the publisher at the address given or the author at the following website.

Author's website: www.praywithderry.com

ISBN-13: 978-1-62652-069-1
LCCN: 2013904924

Cover design by Kristen Bresse

Printed in the United States of America

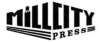

This "quick reference guide" is dedicated to

all that long to make a difference in the lives of those suffering,

and

to all that desire to be effective in hospital ministry.

Table of Contents

Acknowledgments

This handbook, a "quick guide" for effective hospital visitation, is actually the joint effort of a number of people. Unfortunately, I have no idea who all to give credit to because so many have invested in me since I began this journey. But...I will start with the Lord, who called me into this ministry and guided me through every challenge.

Thank you Jesus for trusting me to serve Your people. Thank You for orchestrating so many events in my life to bring this book to fruition. Thank you for all the people You have blessed me with to support and encourage this journey.

With deep appreciation, I acknowledge Sierra Nevada Memorial Hospital, in Grass Valley, CA, where over fifteen years ago I began my career as a Hospital Chaplain. Thank you to the Leadership Team for allowing me to do my internship there and entrusting me to develop a Business Plan Proposal to establish a Chaplain Service Department. Thank you to the Board of Directors for their approval to add spiritual care to our community hospital. Thank you to my Clinical Pastoral Education Supervisor, Rev. Timothy Little, from UC Davis Medical Center in Sacramento, CA, who invested endless hours training, encouraging, and mentoring me.

Shortly after being offered full time employment and accepting the challenge of founding the first Chaplain Service Department at Sierra Nevada, I was asked to establish a volunteer team. It was that request that launched my search for training material. Chaplain Managers and Directors from many hospitals, from all over the United States, came to my rescue and sent their material. With their generous resources came permission to reprint and utilize it as necessity called and opportunities arose. Their material was profound and succinct. The only thing that was lacking on each page was the name of the chaplain or the facility. Consequently, when I put my program together, pulling out material here and there appropriate to my needs from this overwhelming number of submissions, I lost track of who sent what. At that time, it was not a concern since all had given me permission to copy or rewrite anything that would be useful for my training program. But today, I wish I could identify the sources and publicly express my gratitude to each donor.

My heart is anxious to bless our pastors, hospital visitors and our patients with what I have learned. As I review my resources, I cannot but look back to all of the people that poured into me, shared their information, concepts, expertise, and notes of encouragement. Some of you, I have met. Some of you, I may never meet. Nevertheless, thank you for sharing, for covering me with prayer and for helping mold me into the Chaplain that I have become that I might also impart to others.

So how did this book come about and who do I owe most sincere acknowledgements too? Here is the story in sequence:

Over ten years ago now, one of my volunteers, Pam Jung, joined my excitement about writing a training syllabus for chaplain volunteers. From that discussion evolved the desire to create a "cheat sheet" or "checklist" for pastors, spiritual leaders and other hospital visitors to help precipitate an effective and respectful visitation of our patients. Life circumstances caused our idea and material to be shelved.

Early this year, God started nudging me to get this manuscript completed and into the hands of those who can benefit from it. One situation after another has set in motion the completion of this book. It all began again with my dear friend Jeanette Behrmann, emphatically stating, "You need to write a book."

In Spring of 2012, my husband and I took a trip to Florida. Each evening we would go down by the beach and watch the sunset. I started taking pictures. One evening I was able to capture the beautiful sunset shown on the front cover. Brilliant rays of sunshine exuded from a cloud, pointing both toward heaven and toward earth. I expressed that to my husband Ron. When he looked at it, he said, "Maybe you should change the title of your book to: 'Heaven Touches Earth through Hospital Ministry'." That was just what I was thinking! So with the help of my husband, the cover and title emerged along with the continued development of the actual manuscript.

A week later, at a farewell party, I met Kristen Bresse who does layout and design. She suggested that if I would send her the picture, she could design a book cover so that I could prepare handouts and pre-order forms for distribution at the upcoming Association of Professional Chaplains annual conference. She came up with a lovely cover using my sunset picture from Florida.

Our friend, Pastor Darin Shaw, showed up at the house and set to work creating a remarkable first web page for me. Within a few hours, I had acquired a post office box, new business phone number, and a website address to submit to Kristen in time for the printing of the handouts. Since then, Darin has spent an unbelievable amount of time building up social networking and a following for me.

At the chaplain's conference, I sensed God directing me to discuss this book with my friend and colleague, Chaplain Shari Chamberlain. Already having blessed my life in numerous ways, she added to my gratitude by accepting the challenge of editing my manuscript. Her insight and contribution has been a monumental blessing. She often put her own life on hold to accommodate my needs and deadlines. She did an incredible job wading through my manuscript and offering suggestions to enhance its readability and effectiveness. Shari is a gifted teacher, mentor and encourager. I respect her for her integrity and straight-forwardness. I am not only thankful for all she has invested in this book, but also for all that she invests in others, building up her colleagues professionally. To Shari for your unselfish and dependable service, I give deep appreciation.

I also give thanks for other unexpected blessings which arrived in various forms. Like Chaplain Juanita Bartel's Spiritual Wellness, Age Related Chart that I came across. With her permission, I have incorporated some of her findings. Then there is Dorothy Flannery, who by God's design, "just happened" to overhear a discussion I was having with Lynn Ortel about marketing this book. Thank you Lynn for your suggestions and thank you Dorothy for going to work preparing mailing labels and getting email information together for me. Thanks also to Pastor Ray McDaid for his interest, encouragement and suggestions.

The last step of this journey was stumbling across Mark Levine's book, 'The Fine Print of Self Publishing'. After reading his book, I gained direction from a private consultation with him. He and his staff at Mill City Press have been incredible mentors and patient teachers and guides. With their encouragement, feelings of overwhelm and defeat were turned to hopeful anticipation.

It is with much appreciation for all of the effort of those that walked before me, and to all that have walked beside me, that I present this compilation. To each of you, I give big hugs of gratitude. It is my hope that this book will honor those who have shared, those that utilize the contents, and the recipients of your care.

Forward

I am profoundly honored and pleased to have the opportunity to contribute these words of endorsement for the excellent and inspirational handbook, "Heaven Touches Earth Through Hospital Ministry" written by my former student Derry James-Tannariello. I am sure I share with many professors and mentors a deep sense of veneration and joy when former students make contact expressing enthusiasm of their ministry.

While I am learning to become more comfortable with retirement, I look back with sincere gratitude for the more than forty years I was privileged to serve God in ministry. I reflect on the patients, their family members, friends and hospital staff, as well as for my many Clinical Pastoral Education students in Iowa, Georgia and California that I had the opportunity to serve. This ministry has been much more than a job, it has been a life-calling. It is a privilege to have this opportunity to support the ministry of Derry James-Tannariello and to endorse her new book.

As Derry suggests, this is a "handbook" with very practical and "down to earth" suggestions. I would find it helpful in training volunteers, parish visitors and pastors who have not had any Clinical Pastoral Education. As a convenient refresher guide for those who have studied hospital ministry, it is more than a list of do's and don'ts. Derry gives clear insight into hospital protocol and practices to prepare the mind and heart for hospital visitation. The information shared in these pages is punctuated with dramatic stories offered in a spirit of divine inspiration. Derry is a dedicated chaplain who speaks from a heart that is the center of her profound relationship with her Lord. She offers practical advice within a deeply felt spirit. I invite you to be attentive to these practical suggestions given in the warmth and deep-seated dedication of this servant of God.

In working with students, there were probably two themes that I often offered. The first mantra was: "Risk." I encouraged students to risk new possibilities, new ideas, and new experiences. "Behold the turtle who only makes progress when he/she sticks its neck out." The second mantra was: "Show up and shut up." Now that may seem a little over the top, but what I am suggesting is the importance of seeing a pastoral visit as a special time to be <u>present</u> with the patient and their family. Being there to hear deeply, and honor the other is the focus of our ministry. This is not a time to show off our own importance or to get tangled up in our own agendas. Certainly there are words that need to be spoken and Derry suggests many very wise words, but the focus is to be present, and let the spirit of God work for the benefit of the patient and their family members.

I encourage you to approach this handbook with a spirit of enthusiasm. Discover the enlightened truths that are shared here, allowing your ministry to be enriched by these pearls of wisdom.

Reverend Timothy H. Little, DMin., B.C.C., Retired Hospital Chaplain
A.C.P.E. Supervisor and A.A.P.C. Pastoral Counselor

*THE REVEREND DR. TIMOTHY H. LITTLE
DMin. B.C.C. A.C.P.E. Supervisor, A.A.P.C. Pastoral
Counselor. Chaplain Timothy Little recently retired
from more than 40 years of active service in healthcare
ministry, CPE supervision and spiritual counseling.
He has been active in providing leadership in the
Association of Mental Health Clergy, the American
Association of Pastoral Counselors, the Association for
Clinical Pastoral Education as well as the Association
of Professional Chaplains. Most recently he completed
more than 12 years as Certification Chair for Area 13
and 14 covering California, Arizona, Hawaii, Nevada,
and Utah. Chaplain Little was significant in helping
to merge the A.M.H.C. and the College of Chaplains
to form the Association of Professional Chaplains.
Of significant importance to Chaplain Little is his
commitment to his church as a member of the leadership
team of the Presbyterian Association of Specialized
Pastoral Ministries, a Network of the Presbyterian
Health, Education and Welfare Association as well as
his persistent leadership in healthcare issues within his
local Presbytery.*

Introduction

One afternoon I was called to the Emergency Room of our hospital. When I arrived, I found that the patient had just died. I met their minister in the hospital corridor. In utter desperation, his words to me were, "I don't know what to do. I've never done this before. Please tell me what to do."

When visiting a patient, I asked if their family pastor had been notified. She responded, "Oh, he doesn't make hospital visits. He can't handle hospitals."

In speaking to a pastor one evening he said, "I feel so uncomfortable coming to the hospital. It's such a foreign environment. I just don't know what to say or do."

These are samples of reoccurring comments that echo through the corridors each month. These are not isolated events. In my fifteen years of hospital chaplaincy, I have heard these words spoken time and time again. My prayer is that this guidebook will enhance your visitation skills and take away your discomfort of the hospital environment.

My own hospital stay increased and rekindled my empathy for our patients and their support visitors. I still remember my reaction when I heard my doctor state emphatically, "I'm checking you into the hospital NOW!" There was no more arguing; no more bargaining. Those words hit me like a lead balloon. My desk was piled high. My calendar was full. Although I felt tired and overwhelmed by the several hats I wore and the numerous responsibilities I had taken on, I didn't have time to be *in* a hospital bed. My job was to visit **not** to be visited. I was hard hit; discouraged, humiliated. How could this be?

With my bag packed, I stopped by the office one last time to see if anything on my desk needed immediate attention or could be handled from my hospital bed. It was difficult to leave my work behind. I had deadlines to meet; reports due. How long would I have to be in here? How would this end up? And what about the patients that I had promised I would revisit?

As I contemplated all I had on my plate, my awareness of our patients' challenges became keen. I had a deeper realization, understanding and empathy. Many of them come in with the same misgivings, pressures, unfinished business, deadlines looming, and concerns.

My next hurdle was that flimsy, revealing hospital gown. It certainly was anything but flattering. I had sympathized with the patients before, now I certainly concurred with their reactions. I worked at this hospital. I didn't want my co-workers to see me dressed like this….or should I say "undressed" like this.

I thought I was the only one that would be nervous. Not so. The hospital staff knew me and wanted to do everything "right". They wanted to serve me well, and I suppose they were also concerned about my opinion of their care. In their nervousness, I got poked a number of times—more than it usually takes them to find a vein. But the truth is, the medical staff generally *are* concerned that they serve *all* of their patients well.

The next morning, I decided to clean up; but I had trouble walking. There was a window in my door. Hmmm, no privacy. How could I get cleaned up and changed? What if a visitor showed up in the middle of me changing? I limped out of bed and hid in the corner, to tend to my needs.

Settled in now, I waited….and waited….and waited! Waited for what? Anything! I was waiting for a word of what was next, for visitors, for the knowing that I would not be disturbed for awhile so I could take a nap, for test results. I waited and wondered… just like every other patient. Now I could appreciate even more why meal time is so meaningful to our patients. And then, guess what? That's when visitors show up…when my meal is hot, and I am hungry. Visitors come in, and without consideration won't let me eat.

Visitors not trained in hospital etiquette stand in the glare of the window so it's hard to see them. They talk and laugh loud and wear you out asking too many questions and they stay too long. They knock into your medical equipment and "accidentally" hook your IV line.

Where was *my* chaplain? Where was *my* pastor?

Many pastors, many visitors, don't know what to do. They actually do come in and walk all over the tubing, stand in a glare, or sit on the bed. They don't think of the importance of checking in with the medical staff before entering your room or even of calling ahead and checking to see if you will be available. They might come and find you away, out getting medical tests, asleep, or worse yet—in a mess. In their anxiety to minister a blessing, there are so many small things that they are unaware of, or forget about, that might make a difference in the effectiveness of their visit. That is another reason for this book.

Many clergy feel out of their comfort zone when visitation of a parishioner is needed. If that is how you feel, you're certainly not alone. Part of my role as a chaplain is to serve the religious community by providing relevant experience and support, and to enable our spiritual leaders to minister effectively to their hospitalized parishioners and friends. Whether pastor or hospital visitor, my wish is to help you feel as comfortable and "in charge" at a hospital facility, as you are ministering anywhere else.

When we are uncomfortable in a situation, or it is a new experience, we often do not even know what questions to ask in order to equip ourselves for a positive outcome. This *easy to follow handbook* is complete with check lists (or cheat sheets) that will give you guidelines in ministering in various situations. This step by step guide will answer some of your unasked questions and provide you with tools to help generate a successful and supportive visit and increase your confidence when your ministry takes you to the foreign environment of a healthcare facility. Carry it with your Bible so you can sneak a peek when confronted with the unknown or unexpected.

What a difference it would have made for me had I known when to expect visitors. I wasn't able to rest well during the day because

I was afraid if I closed my eyes and a visitor did come and looked through the window on my door they would think I was asleep. I would miss them.

What a difference it would have made had I been allowed to eat my meal while it was hot. After all, I had waited all morning. It was uncomfortable for me to eat in front of them and even when the nurse came in to take away my tray and realized I hadn't eaten yet; even though I stated outright that I didn't want to eat in front of them, they didn't pick up on it and give me a few minutes.

What a difference it would have made if they had just come to the other side of my bed instead of standing in the glare. What a difference it would have made if they hadn't jostled me or pulled my IV line. That hurt!

My desire is that after you visit, the staff, as well as the patient, rather than wishing that you had shortened your visit, or dreading the next visit, will be left with a blessing. They will have a deep sense of gratitude for your hospital etiquette and respect of hospital regulations, for your thoughtfulness and courtesy, and for your ministry to the patient's specific needs with compassionate care.

Visitation Etiquette

Hospital visits can be uplifting and encouraging, or embarrassing and demoralizing as the following story quoted from page 180 of "The Healing Power of Humor" by Allen Klein, relates. This story was recounted by a middle-aged male pastor.

I had a very serious accident a few years ago; it was amazing I survived. And, of course, I was in the hospital for a very long time recuperating. Because I was there for so long, I became rather nonchalant with the nurses about the procedures they subjected me to—you can't keep decorum up for very long with no clothes on. I was also having trouble finding a relatively painless spot to put yet another injection of pain medication… One time I rang for the nurse, and when she came on the intercom, I told her I needed another pain shot. I knew it would take just about as long for her to draw up the medication as it would for me to gather the strength to roll over and find a spot for her to inject it. I had succeeded in rolling over, facing away from the door, when I heard her come in. "I think this area here isn't too bad," I said, pointing to an exposed area of my rear. But there was an awful silence after I said that. My face paled as I rolled over slowly to see who had actually come in –it was one of my twenty-two year old female parishioners! I apologized and tried to chat with her, but she left shortly thereafter, horribly embarrassed."

In this particular case, it was a pastor that was the patient. Both patient and visitor was embarrassed. How can we avoid participating in an embarrassing moment? Let's look together at how to prepare and work through a visit from beginning to end. In this chapter, we will cover:

- The Definition of a Visit
- Touch
- Preparation for the Visit
- Caring Communication
- When You Arrive at the Hospital
- Disruptions to Caring Communication
- Entering Room
- Calling the Nurse
- The Visit
- When Family Members are Present
- Posturing
- Concluding the Visit

Definition of "visit": Visit according to Webster means "to go and see for the purpose of giving comfort and aid". A "good" visit should comfort, nourish, inspire, instruct, befriend, and enhance relationships.

WHY VISIT?

- The potential for healing of the patient is increased.
- You represent the presence of God and church community in the midst of illness, suffering, and human need.
- Being visited offers breakthrough to the hospitalized in their isolation and loneliness.
- When the patient is visited they feel valued.
- Sometimes it is to meet the expectations of the patient, family, or hospital personnel, prior to surgery or during emergencies.
- A visit may rectify strained relations. (You may not have a favorable relationship with the patient. Remember that agape love doesn't require that you like the person; however you are required to forgive and "love your neighbor as yourself.")

Incorporating hospital etiquette, understanding the patient's needs and applying appropriate pastoral tools while ministering in a healthcare facility, will give you the confidence to focus on your relationship and support of your hospitalized parishioner.

To prevent burdensome communication, I will be using the term "patient" interchangeably. "Patient" can refer to the person actually hospitalized, one suffering from illness, or the one placed before you that needs your ministering attention. This could be a family member, friend, caregiver or a member of the medical staff.

One of our most vulnerable times, in life, is when we are hospitalized. It is a time when we are most prone to heart searching and begin questioning life after death. It is also a time when a pastor can most effectively talk to a patient where they are suffering spiritually, because the patient is most open. This is a time when family members might try to "bargain" with God to intervene for the patient. A discerning pastor will utilize these opportunities without taking undue advantage of the patient by leading him/her into a conversation that they are not yet prepared to take part in. This is a time that the pastor needs keen sensitivity, respect and patience.

Issues of forgiveness, after life, God's grace and peace, are all subjects that may need to be explored with the patient. Unresolved forgiveness issues cause stress that sets the body up for disease. Walk cautiously, but boldly, under the anointing of the Holy Spirit.

PREPARATION FOR THE VISIT

1. Take business cards or note cards with you to leave on the bedside table if the patient is sleeping or out of the room.

2. PRAY, PRAY, PRAY and did I mention Pray? Inviting God to precede you will prepare the patient for your visit. When you are prayed up, and walking in His empowerment, God will anoint your lips and give you discernment to zone in on the patient's deepest heart need.

3. Ask yourself:
    A. "Why am I going?"
    *   Am I going for the purpose of giving comfort and aid or for socializing?
    *   Am I going out of duty or curiosity? If the answer is duty—adjust your attitude.
    *   If you are resisting the visit, figure out why and address it with God.

B. **"How is my own health?"**

- Don't go if you are sick yourself. This is for your precaution as well as for patient and staff. You jeopardize the patient's health further—and could endanger a new baby.
- If you do have to go while you are sick, go to the nurse's station and ask for a mask.
- The alternative is to use the phone. In this case, it would certainly be more honoring to pray over the phone.

C. **"What are the visiting hours and number of visitors allowed in the room at a time?"**

- You don't want to be there during bath, bathroom check, dressing changes, medical interventions, or when they are out for procedures or scheduled tests. If visiting new moms, not when they are nursing baby.
- When you say that you're coming—Come!

D. **"What time is surgery?"**

- Make your visit before surgery so that you can have prayer with them and if possible stay during surgery so that you can be with the family.
- According to one doctor-If you think that the surgery is minor, consider that anytime a surgeon picks up his knife, and the anesthesiologist is called—it is serious.
- Families need comforting. Sometimes they are terrified. The doctor says an hour or two, so when it goes on for three or four hours, their imagination goes wild. Your presence would bring a sense of calm. This is when your presence is really appreciated. The clock seems to tick slowly.

4. Dress like a visitor—simple and casual.
   - Not like you are ready to conduct a funeral. (It can terrify the patient.)
   - Avoid wearing anything with a fragrance, i.e. after-shave lotion, cologne, deodorant, or hair spray. **(Fragrances can cause or increase nausea.)**
   - For a considerable period of time prior to your visit, don't smoke or come from a place where people have been smoking.
   - Wear closed toe shoes (for own protection).

5. Come as a friend—that just happens to be a spiritual representative vs coming as a pastor <u>over</u> the parishioner. Jesus was all about relationship. He is our example.

6. Be emotionally prepared for anything so you are not surprised by the unexpected, i.e. patient's appearance, odors, attitudes, lack of mobility, itching, disorientation, or confessions. If you feel uncomfortable or uneasy, it may have negative repercussions and be damaging to your ministry.
   - Don't be insulted by the patient's attitude. They are medicated, in pain, scared, mad at everybody. They might say and do things that will totally embarrass you. These should never be mentioned outside the room to anyone.
   - Show genuine concern and respect.
   - Do not compare patients, previously or present.

7. Consider age and developmental stage

• Infant	Trust	Move slowly
• Toddler	Autonomy	Encourage their capabilities
• Preschooler	Imagination	Interested in listening
• School Age	Industry	Bring puzzles or word games
• Adolescent	Identity	Choose words carefully. Patient maybe self-conscious, embarrassed or overly sensitive.
• Young Adult	Intimacy	Loved ones are important
• Middle-Aged	Generativity	Concern over financial pressures. How will we make it through this?
• Elderly	Integrity	Focus is family reconciliation and after life issues

WHEN YOU ARRIVE AT THE HOSPITAL

- Park in a proper parking place; not in restricted areas. Look for clergy designated parking spots for your use. Think of yourself as part of the hospital staff.

- Stop and pray. Recommit this visit and request wisdom to impart according to the needs of the patient and their family members.

- Go to Information Desk in the hospital lobby to verify room number, get directions and introduce yourself. Sometimes patients are moved from room to room. It is prudent to check each time prior to the visit. It will save embarrassment as well as an interruption to the nursing staff.

- Some facilities provide identification badges. If you have one, wear it so that in an emergency you are easily identified and included in the healthcare team.

- If not, check at the Information Desk, Spiritual Care Department, or Human Resources, to see if they provide clergy ID badges.

- On the way to the patient's room, remember to speak softly in consideration of other patients along the way. This is not the time for loud talking, laughing or joking. Avoid participating in such, even with staff.

- Check in at Nursing Station. Introduce/identify yourself and ask if it is an appropriate time to visit your parishioner in room #_____. Ask how ill they are before going in. Ask if they have expressed any spiritual needs or struggles.

- They will not be able to give you specifics on their disease or diagnosis, but can tell you whether they are conscious or sleeping, have a fever, etc. Ask the nurse if it is okay to awaken the patient if they are asleep. Some units, such as Intensive Care, have specific regulations (like no flowers) so it is imperative you inquire at the Nursing Station of <u>each</u> unit.

- Infection control: Always make sure you wash your hands before you go into the room and as you are leaving. The best infection control for you and the patient is proper hand hygiene.
- Safety: Just before you walk in the door, look over the door and see if the light is on. If it is, do not enter. Read and observe **all** signs that are on the door.

    No visitors--Do not enter--check at the Nurse's Station

    Isolation--gown or mask (A cart will be outside of patient's door with supplies.)

    Oxygen in use--**This means caution!** Don't bring in things that can spark or burn. **Why?**

Ex: Parents brought their son a birthday cake, and opened the oxygen tent for him to blow out the candles. The party turned to tragedy. The child was blown up.

Ex: A gentleman who used an electric shaver while wearing an oxygen mask faced the same tragedy.

ENTERING ROOM *(Be prepared for odors)*

- Turn off cell phone and put it away. You are there for the patient. This is their time—a sacred appointment.
- Respect pulled curtains. Remember you are entering someone's temporary bedroom: personal space. Patients may be dressing or have messed themselves. If they are extremely embarrassed by your visit they might not return to church. Wait until the situation has been handled.
- Always knock softly so as not to wake the sleeping patient, unless you have received permission from the

nurse. Ask, "May I come in?" Some patients will be extremely disappointed if you don't awaken them and they miss your visit. (Patients are awakened by the nursing staff at regular intervals to check their vitals. Hospitals are not the place to come if you want rest.)

- First impressions important—observe items in room—card, flowers, balloons, stuffed animals for conversation starters.
- Be positive.
- Enter, listening for the voice of suffering.

THE VISIT

Remember that patients don't need to hear bad reports…yours or anyone else's…including the national news. They already have enough problems just to recover. Don't torture them with horror stories. ("I know how you feel. My friend had the same thing, and she died." Or "I had a friend that had the same thing and he's paralyzed. He never did get over it.") Reserve making any comments regarding medication and all health care. Uplifting stories and positive communication promote hope and health.

Beware of giving too much sympathy. Some patients thrive on it. Ask yourself, "What can I do for this patient? They have a doctor watching over their health, nurses checking on them regularly tending their needs, meals prepared and delivered, and Environmental Services cleaning their room. What can I do for them?"

If they talk—listen. They need and deserve your <u>complete</u> attention. If they need encouragement—support them. So begin the visit…

- The assumption is that by now, you are prayed up and ready…right?

- Clarify who you are if there seems to be any confusion.
- Leave your business card or note if they are asleep.
- Respect other patients in the room. Acknowledge their presence. (God may have sent you there for them too.)
- Be aware of your noise level.
- Upon entrance, scrutinize patient. Are they happy to see you? Are they depressed, teary, listless, anxious, weak, in pain? How is their breathing? How is their color? Flushed, yellow, blue?
- Leave almost immediately if the patient is in pain, has nausea, or bowel/urinary problems.
- Avoid standing in front of a window where the glare could cause discomfort for the patient. Don't sit, lean on or bump patient's bed. You might cause much pain.
- Do not place your personal items on the empty bed. It is sanitized and ready for the next patient.
- Leave the room at mealtime so they can eat while it is hot. Don't eat off the patient's tray.
- Leave the room if a nurse or doctor comes in. Doctor sometimes only comes in once a day. Patient may want to ask some personal questions and is embarrassed to ask you to step out, or ask in front of you. They might well need answers. Just say, "I'll step out and get a drink of water and be right back."
- Don't ever follow the doctor out the door and talk (whisper) within ear shot.
- Don't whisper. The patient may think you are discussing something about them that they are not yet informed about. They may think they are not being told the whole truth. **Even if they are in a coma or asleep, they can hear.** If the patient knows that the doctor and the pastor are

whispering...(s)he may think he is in serious trouble, and that something is critically wrong. Wait until you are at a private place to carry on your conversation. Bits of conversation may be overheard, misinterpreted and cause alarm.

- Make visits brief in an unhurried way. (15 minutes at the most. Five minutes being best unless they have serious issues they need to discuss.) Don't hurry the person being visited. Work with them at their own pace. Let them share without interrogating them with multiple questions.
- Don't assume that just because the patient is facing discharge and going home that he/she is happy.
  - Maybe they don't have the money for the operation they need.
  - Maybe there is no place they hate more than home. There could be relationship problems, or their home is uncomfortable or dirty.
  - Maybe they were enjoying it at the hospital. It is the only place where they have had any attention, freedom from pain, care or socializing.

POSTURING—SITTING HELPS THEM RELAX

- Pick a place to sit (or stand if necessary) that is directly in the place of eye contact with the patient; but:
  - **not** in front of an open window or light. Light glaring in patient's eyes could cause a headache, hurt their eyes or make them uncomfortable.
  - **not** on patient's bed, or any other bed in the room even if nobody is in it.
- If you sit on patient's bed, you might accidentally cause them pain or discomfort, or bring in outside germs—

one more thing to tax their immune system. Any vacant bed has already been sanitized and is ready for a new patient. **Do not** place any items on it.

- Don't make patient turn or change positions.
- Watch for **equipment** around the room and **cords/ tubes** on the floor. Some visitors are curious as to how the equipment works. **Do not touch!**

Story: One dear pastor confessed he has trouble keeping his hands off of any mechanical equipment and began investigating. He touched where he shouldn't have touched and the alarms went off. Another visitor was so nervous about visiting in the hospital that he didn't realize he was standing on the tubing on the floor cutting off patient's support.

TOUCH—PHYSICAL TOUCH IS REASSURING AND COMMUNICATES CARING

- Ask before you reach out to touch/take hand unless the patient extends hand. The patient might have a dislocated shoulder or some other injured area that you could cause pain to. Touch their arm gently.
- Appropriate touch and/or touch with permission can be welcome, affirming, healing, and comforting. A simple, light touch on the arm, hand or shoulder should be natural and spontaneous.
- One must be careful not to cross boundaries here. Sensitivity is required.
- Hold hands during prayer.

CARING COMMUNICATION

We think of communication as "speaking" and "listening". In hospital ministry we expand that understanding. "Speaking" consists of three parts: facts, thoughts and feelings. "Listening" includes complete attention, presence, body language and <u>hearing with your heart</u> the voice of suffering.

Strengthen relationships by showing respect and genuine acceptance, exuding warmth and compassionate caring, building rapport and promising confidentiality. Enter into the patient's world. Look beyond the surface, beyond their words, to their deepest point of suffering. Are they fearful of upcoming diagnosis or procedures? Are they worried about how this hospitalization will affect their family, their relationships, their job, or their future?

Put yourself in their shoes and try to look at things from their perspective. Be aware of your own feelings and prejudices so that they will not interfere with your relationship with the patient or your ministry to them.

Talk easily, without feeling pressured. Be natural and relaxed. Don't make the patient feel as if they have to host or entertain you.

Suggestions:
- Be in a good mood. Be positive. Share some joy. Be brief.
- Being too jovial and causing the post surgical patient to laugh could create pain and possible complications. Be thoughtful even in your humor.
- Warm, caring tone of voice, facial expressions, and body language all speak volumes to patients.
- Voice should be calming, peaceful, understanding, caring, empathetic.

- Turn toward patient to indicate full attention.
- Lean towards them. (approx. 3 feet)
- Be attentive and relaxed. Nod your head.
- Have eye contact (expressive eyes), raise eyebrows.
- Smile. Use facial expressions showing interest, concern or understanding.
- Use their name and make positive, encouraging statements about them.
- Talk about subjects that are familiar and meaningful to patient.
- Let the patient choose the course of the conversation.
- **Be a skilled listener.** Be sensitive to their anxiety, discomfort, or embarrassment. Patient should be given the opportunity to do most of the talking. Respond with— "hmm, oh". Interrupt only to clarify information.
- Reflect their feelings. Some patients are afraid to share their true feelings for fear they will project weakness or lack of faith. They pretend to be strong and courageous. If you detect them doing this, give them permission to release their feelings.
- Statements like "I care about you; about how you're holding up." or "I'm concerned about you." or "Tell me what's going on with you." All will provide patient the opportunity to share whatever they want about their condition. (Informational questions can pull them away from feelings they need to discuss and work through.)
- If ever there was a time to be an attentive listener, it is when you are visiting in the hospital. Sometimes total silence is even more appreciated. Your presence and a gentle touch can make all the difference. Listen with your heart for the voice of suffering and a desire to understand.

- Evaluate the patient's remarks. "Why are they telling me this right now?" "What might they want from me?—Resources? Affirmations?" "What are their needs, conflicts, concerns, fears, strengths?"
- Watch for verbal and non-verbal clues.
- Avoid telling them how they feel, like "I know you must be in terrible pain."
- Question "How are things going?" Rather than "How do you feel?" Patient has been reading, watching TV, sleeping, trying to take their mind off of how they feel, and then we come in and ask them how they feel. (Be prepared for criticism of the hospital.)
- Be extremely aware of people's feelings and attitudes. Reflect on feelings and the issues presented.
- Denial is a vital defense. If it is strong, don't attempt to counter it. Give patient opportunity to work through it.
- Possible feelings you might encounter are: fear, loneliness, uncertainty, anxiety, anger, irritability, depression, guilt, boredom, apathy, sadness, confusion, disorientation, paranoia, discomfort, or embarrassment.
- Possible physical conditions might be: pain, nausea, itching, weakness, thirst, lack of mobility.
- Express empathy by acknowledging the feelings they have been sharing.
- Use "I feel" statements. "I'm sorry." (Genuine caring).
- Reflect back—accepting their feelings and sharing your perceptions, inviting them to explore the situation with you and clarify the issues. Neither agree nor disagree. (Reflections are **not** interpretations.)
- Repeat key words. Ask open questions.
- Summarize/Paraphrase: Integrate their feelings. Do not give solutions.

- Affirm trust in them to solve their own problem with God's help. Find something genuinely positive to say.
- Don't be drawn into criticism, impatience, or irritation. Some patients want to criticize everybody--the doctors, the nurse, the food. This is typical of people with medical problems given the situation they are in. If you're not careful you'll get lured right into it. Never criticize the institution. Try to reassure them that they are in a safe place. Suggest that perhaps the staff member was just distracted or had a particularly difficult day full of emergencies or unexpected challenges. This will help the patient feel more secure and perhaps relieve their own fears and questions. Older people are particularly sensitive to criticism.
- Be understanding and encouraging if the patient seems apathetic spiritually. Patient might not even want to pray. They may question or be angry with God.
- Respect their views and their right to make their own decisions.
- What do you say when the patient asks, "Why is this happening to me?" Respond, "I don't know." Don't try to have all the answers. Present Jesus as the perfect example of suffering. He didn't rebel against it or try to escape it. He faced it. Walk with them in search of meaning.
- Ask if they have any particular scripture that is meaningful to them. (Psalms 23, Romans 8, John 14, Psalms 137:1-4) See the chapter on Healing Scriptures.
- Do not offer false optimism or try to predict the outcome contrary to what the doctors are saying, or comment on the medication patient is taking. We all want to be hopeful, but we also need to be realistic. (This does not mean that we cannot exercise prayer and faith, according to God's will.)

- Don't appear to the patient as a "faith healer" making demands of God for the removal of suffering and disease, or building false hope.
- You do not know God's will for this particular patient.
- You do not know if they have violated laws of health or if they are harboring unforgiveness which has caused this health crises.
- Your declarations can be devastating to the faith of the patient, their trust in you, and their view of their value to God if God doesn't answer in the way you have requested/demanded.
- Appeal to God for them to have courage and strength, peace and grace in the midst of this health challenge/crises.
- Ask God to reveal ways that they could better care for their body temple in the future.
- Pray God's promises according to His destiny for them.
- Instill a sense of God's love and presence.
- Comfort the patient with the hope and assurance we have in Christ now and eternally.
- Pray for them and their family. Your prayer and loving concern will create an atmosphere where the love and presence of God are felt and the Holy Spirit can minister.

Story: Even after hospice was involved, the church group came over and told the patient "You'll be out of here in a few days." In this case, the doctors were coming in and trying to prepare her for death and this group was doing just the opposite.

If you've heard the prognosis is death, the patient and the family might still be in denial. An appropriate question might be: "How do you feel about your condition?"

Story: The pastor came in and told the patient, "You'll be alright in a few days." The doctor came in a few days later and told her that she had terminal cancer and tried to prepare her for the inevitable. She was mad.

People feel like you, as a pastor, are a representative of God and that whatever you say is a message from God to them. She felt God must have been lying to promise her hope. Be careful about offering false optimism.

- **Prayer**--Having faith and praying for people to get well is something else entirely. We could say something like, "Thank God we still have prayer." or God's word says He will be our guide even unto death and His plan for each of us is to live with Him forever; so we will pray that the enemy's plans are thwarted and God's destiny for you will be fulfilled. As we trust in Him, we can be thankful that no one can interrupt that perfect plan. He holds your future. He alone knows. We will continue to pray for healing according to God's plan for your eternal salvation, but we know that **"Healing is not always cure."** Leave soon after prayer so that words spoken to God in patient's behalf will be left foremost in their thoughts.

- **Keep Confidences**-everything shared should remain in that room. Remember that everything that is told to you is entirely confidential. The nurses take a pledge called a Nightingale pledge, where he/she vows before man and God, "I will hold in confidence all personal matters committed to my keeping, all family affairs coming to my knowledge in the practice of my profession." Essentially, doctors have the same pledge. We should do it too. We should never discuss one person with another.

HIPPA laws protect patient privacy and metes out large fines in violation of breached confidentiality. Often people in the hospital think they are dying, and decide to make confessions that would not be made under other circumstances. Many serious confessions from way back in the past are made in the last two weeks of life.

Ex. "Pastor, I'm not trying to be negative, but if anything happens to me—I have another child that no one knows anything about, and I want to see that the child is taken care of."

Whatever is said is highly confidential and must not be discussed. There are exceptions: If the patient expresses a desire to hurt oneself or others, this must be reported to appropriate people.

DISRUPTIONS TO CARING COMMUNICATION

- Facial or body language showing shock, judgment, distain or rejection
- Diverting, avoiding, changing the subject, or withdrawing
- Kidding, teasing, using sarcasm
- Dealing with facts and not feelings
- Questioning, probing
- Warning, advising or offering solutions without patient requesting your opinion
- Disagreeing or criticizing their decisions
- Shaming them by passing judgment, promoting guilt or putting them down with a laugh
- Interpreting or psychoanalyzing
- Talking about yourself or sharing your story

- Comparing or talking about someone else's experience and responses
- Repeating confidential matters about another person
- Look at your watch, or somewhere else: out the window. Not focused on speaker
- Checking or fiddling with your cell phone, clean fingernails or glasses
- Close your eyes, yawn
- Open your book or newspaper, crossword, Sudoku

CALL THE NURSE TO ADDRESS PATIENT'S NEEDS
- Don't change the patient's position or adjust bed; though an innocent gesture, it may be to the patient's detriment.
- Don't give them water. They might be off liquids in order to prepare for surgery or water might make them nauseous.
- Don't alter air vents or adjust temperature. Avoid comments like "Wow, I'm too cold in here." *[You might bring a jacket. Hospital rooms are deliberately cool to retard the growth of germs]*
- If patient voices complaints, pass them on to a nurse, if appropriate.
- Do not try to settle problems beyond the scope of your position or training. You are not expected to be a social worker, a chaplain, a doctor, or a lawyer.

WHEN FAMILY MEMBERS ARE PRESENT:
- Make family members as much a part of your ministry as patient. Sometimes the family is more distraught than the patient.

- Be aware of and attentive to their needs.
- Assist them with decision-making by letting them talk through it finding their own solution. Encourage them to talk to pertinent medical advisors.

CONCLUDING THE VISIT

- Be sure patient has a dependable support team; if not, engage the congregation.
- Knowing the patient's spirituality and faith belief is beneficial. Read encouraging scripture or other inspirational material.
- They may not know whether this is a routine visit to show you care and want to encourage them or if you know something they don't and you are there to break bad news and administer a "death prayer". Reassure them.
- Offer to pray for them before you leave, but say something like, "Would you like for me to pray for you now, or would you rather I remember you later in private prayer?" Some people would rather you do it later. They might be dealing with issues of fear, disorientation, or other personal concerns that they are not ready to discuss. Ask what they would like you to include in the prayer for them personally. Leave shortly thereafter so remembrance of blessing will remain with them.
- Keep promises. Be careful what you promise. Don't promise to come back to the hospital without forethought. If you say that you are going to come at a certain time, be there. Patient has nothing else to do but watch the clock and wait for you. Leave yourself room for delay. The patient may go from upset to mad if you

are late. They may want to nap and are holding off until you leave. They may expend reserve energy to clean up for you. You can say something like, "I'd like to say that I'll see you tomorrow at 2:00, but since I often have unexpected things come up, I'll have to say, I'll try my best to see you at that time. If I find I am unable to come, I will call and let you know."

- Ask permission to put them on the prayer line at church and ask if they need help with transporting children, having meals delivered at home, or any other support. Let them know you will be thinking about them and praying for them.
- Wash your hands.

Hospital Protocol Summary

Preparation for the visit:
- Ask yourself: "Why am I going?"
- Ask yourself: "How is my own health?"
- Ask yourself: "What are the visiting hours?"
- When you say that you're coming—come. Be on time.
- Find out: What time surgery is and how much before that you should come. Plan to stay with the family. *(Confirm by phone call before coming, as times change.)*
- Be emotionally prepared for anything—patient's appearance, attitudes, confessions, smell.

When you arrive at the hospital:
- Park in a proper parking place.
- Leave any of your negative or troubled emotions outside the hospital. Positive emotions such as compassion, peacefulness, etc. are effective.
- Go to the Information Desk and verify room # and get directions.
- On the way to the patient's room, as well as in the room, remember to speak softly.
- Check in at nurse's station—introduce yourself.
- Always make sure your hands are clean before you go into the room and after you leave.
- Read and observe all signs that are on the door. If the light is on over door, do not enter.
- Always knock.

The Visit:

- If the patient is asleep, let him/her sleep unless you have permission from the nurse to awaken them.
- Leave your card.
- Respect other patients in the room.
- Make visits brief. (15 minutes at the most--5 minutes best unless they have serious issues they need to discuss.) Be mindful of their ability to talk soon after surgery.
- First impressions are important. Observe items in room—cards, flowers, etc. for conversation starters.
- Communicate the purpose of your visit with a loving, positive attitude.
- Listen with your heart and be careful of communication with others in the room.
- Help them address any issues of unforgiveness: to others, God, or self. (This can open them for healing.)
- Keep confidences. Everything shared should remain in that room.
- Ask before you reach out to touch or take their hands, unless the patient extends hand. Touch them gently, or hold their hand during prayer if they like.
- Pick a place to sit or stand that gives you good eye contact with the patient, but **not** in front of an open window or light, and **not** on the beds.
- Be careful and watchful of **equipment** around the room and **cords/tubing** on the floor.
- Respect and cooperate with any hospital employees that come into the room.
- Observe all hospital rules.
- Leave at mealtime or if a doctor or nurse come in.
- Do not follow medical staff or other visitors out the door and whisper in hall.

Concluding Visit:

- Offer to read inspirational thoughts and/or have prayer.
- Leave a written scripture, encouraging thought or inspirational reading material.
- Don't promise to come back at a certain time.
- Let them know you will be thinking of them and praying for them.
- Ask if church family can be notified to pray for and support them.
- Wash your hands.

Environment of Care

HOSPITAL ENVIRONMENT

Hospitals are sterile *and* infected. This is a paradox! On one hand, we may enter the hospital milieu and be immediately met with the smell of disinfectants, and then go into the patient's room and have to resist the urge to plug our nose. We put our hands in our pockets in fear of becoming contaminated and wonder what we're really doing here.

This chapter delineates the precautions needed to protect you, the patient, and others present when visiting at the hospital. In this chapter pertinent information will be presented about:

Warnings-posted on the door of the patient's room

Precautions-to protect yourself and the patient

Codes-indicating emergency needs

Common Medical Abbreviations-hospital terminology

So let's begin:

WARNINGS

It is critical that upon entrance of a patient's room, you look for warnings posted on or outside of their door. These warnings will give specific instructions as to what you should:

- wear…such as gloves, masks, gowns, or protective eye-covering
- not carry into the room

If a supply cart with masks is outside patient's door, check warning signs for your own protection as well as patient's.

If in doubt, BE SURE to check with the nursing station before entering. Typical warnings could be:

Airborne Precautions

AFB Isolation

Contact Precautions

Droplet Precautions

Immunosuppressive Care Precautions

Oxygen In Use

When you see precautionary signs, take time to read them. The explanations and instructions will be clear.

PRECAUTIONS:

As a general rule, if you have open cuts or abrasions on your hands it is wise to wear gloves to protect yourself and the patient. Open sores expose you to the threat of MRSA; an infection so hostile that if not immediately treated could result in amputation. You can help control the spread of infection by:

- Practicing proper personal hygiene
- Discarding any used gloves before leaving room.
- Visiting only if you are well and free of infection
- Washing your hands frequently using appropriate handwashing techniques

    …before and after contact with patient

    …before and after handling any food you might bring patient

    …after using the restroom

    …after touching face, scratching head, blowing nose

Although all of us carry germs on our skin as normal flora, the purpose of hand washing is to remove transient bacteria picked up on our hands from handling patients, objects and touching surfaces.

Proper hand sanitizing:
Hand sanitizing machines are generally spaced throughout the hallway. Be sure and rub liberal amount on front and back of hands and fingers. This technique is easier but not as effective as proper hand washing, described below.

Proper hand washing technique:
- Completely wet hands and wrists under running water
- Apply soap liberally
- Hold your hands lower than your elbows
- Work up a good lather, rubbing between and around fingers, and under and around nail beds using friction for at least 15 seconds
- Rinse well under running water
- Dry thoroughly with paper towels
- Use a paper towel to turn off water. Never touch the faucet with your hands after washing. The faucet is considered contaminated. Throw the paper towel into the wastepaper basket. Avoid touching the basket. **NEVER** push trash down. (You never know if there are infected towels or sharps inadvertently placed in the trash. Ex. Diabetics use sharps to inject insulin.)
- Complete your hand washing with liberal use of hand sanitizer found in the patient's room or in the hallway. If it is not easily available, ask at the nurses' station.
- If a patient has MRSA (Methicillin-resistant Staphylococcus aureus) or CDiff both sanitizer and soap **must be used** to insure your safety.

CODES

If you are a frequent visitor be sure and check the codes at your particular hospital. There are variations at different facilities. Examples of codes that might be used are as follows:

> Code **Amber** – Missing patient/person
> Code **Black** – Bomb Threat
> Code **Blue** – Respiratory Emergency/Cardiac Arrest
>   CPR Adult
> Code **1 or Gray** – Security Alert/Violent/Combative
>   Situation
> Code **Green** -- Evacuation
> Code **Orange** – Disaster/Spill/HazMat Release
> Code **Orange EMS** – Patient(s) Decon
> Code **Orange MSI** – Radioactive Haz Mat
> Code **Pink** – Infant Abduction/Infant Delivery
>   (Not in L&D)
> Code **Purple** – Child Abduction/Surge Capacity
> Code **Red** – Fire (See RACE below)
> Code **Silver** – Weapon/Hostage
> Code **Triage** – Internal or External Emergency
> Code **White** – Respiratory Emergency/CPR Pediatric
> Code **Yellow** – Bomb Threat/Discovery
> **Med. Alert** – Med. Assistance Hosp. Premise

If you are visiting your parishioner, friend or family member and you become aware of a problem, it might be valuable for you to know how to get immediate response. Ask the receptionist what number to dial if an emergency were to occur. Some hospitals have you dial 444, others 2111. State the code or problem and give the location.

Important abbreviations for you to be familiar with would be:

CHD	Coronary heart disease
CHF	Congestive heart failure
CCU	Coronary care unit
DNR	Do not resuscitate
DOA	Dead on arrival
ICU	Intensive Care Unit
NICU	Neo-natal intensive care unit
PICU	Pediatrics Intensive Care Unit
WICU	Women and Infants Care Unit

COMMON MEDICAL ABBREVIATIONS

If you are a chaplain, pastor or hospital visitor in training, the following information may be enlightening and helpful for you as you minister. These abbreviations or terms may be on the white board in the patient's room.

Medical Terms, Abbreviations, and Definitions

ADT	admission, discharge, transfer
AMA	against medical advice
B/P, BP	blood pressure
BID, bid	twice a day
BIN, bin	twice a night
BM	bowel movement
Bx	biopsy
CA	cancer, carcinoma
CABG	coronary artery bypass graft
Cal	calorie
CAT	computerized axial tomography
Cath	catheter
CCU	coronary care unit
Ch	cholesterol
CHB	complete heart block
CHD	coronary heart disease
CHF	congestive heart failure
COPD	chronic obstructive pulmonary disease

D/C, DC	discontinue
disch	discharge
DNR	do not resuscitate
DOA	dead on arrival
DR	delivery room
Dx	diagnosis
ECG/EKG	electrocardiogram
FX, fx	fracture
GI	gastrointestinal
GSW	gunshot wound
GYN, gyn	gynecology
I & D	incision and drainage
I & O	intake and output
ICU	intensive care unit
Incontinent	lacking self-restraint
Isol	isolation
IV	intravenously
L & D	labor and delivery
Lab	laboratory
Lesion	an injury or wound
LPN	licensed practical nurse
MI	myocardial infarction
MRI	magnetic resonance imaging
MRSA	methicillin-resistant staphylococcus aureus
MSCC	medical surgical critical care

NICU	neo-natal intensive care unit
NPO	nothing by mouth
NYD	not yet diagnosed
od	once a day
OPD	outpatient department
Px	prognosis
q2h	every two hours
qd	every day
qh	every hour
QID, qid	four times a day
R/O	rule out
RAT	radiation therapy
rehab	rehabilitation
RN	registered nurse
STAT, stat	immediately
VS	vital signs
WICU	women & infants care unit

Understanding Patient's Needs—Effective Ministry

WHAT YOU NEED TO KNOW ABOUT THE PATIENTS YOU ARE VISITING:

During my stay in the hospital, I remember watching the clock, waiting for my friends to come. I was afraid that if I closed my eyes—even to pray—someone might peek through the window in my door and see me. They would think I was asleep and not come in. If I expected them before a certain time and they didn't arrive, I was disapointed.

There was a sink in the room which was my only means for cleaning up. If anyone peeked in the door, or worse yet, opened the door without knocking or waiting for a response—they would have gotten an eye full and we both would have been embarrassed.

Another time, a day I was particularly hungry and had been waiting for lunch to arrive, a visitor dropped by shortly after my meal had been delivered. Because it was awkward and difficult to eat, I did not feel comfortable eating in front of them. Even though I stated that fact out right, knowing they had other things they could do for a few minutes, they just sat there and droned on and on. The nurse came in to retrieve my tray twice. I kept assuring her that I would eat it after my guest left. A happier visit and a more thoughtful visitor would have excused themselves for about 15 minutes to afford me the opportunity to eat my meal while it was hot.

How does being sick, or worse yet dying, affect patients in the hospital? Try putting yourself in their shoes. Indeed you may have already experienced a hospital stay yourself or have been called in for support.

When a patient and family first hear their diagnosis or prognosis, they rarely 'hear' all of what has been said. A follow-up discussion should take place with their doctor or attending nurse to answer questions, to clear up any misunderstanding or misconstruing of information and assist with clarification. A well-trained and informed pastor in attendance can help minimize denial and shock. It's also important to remember that relapses of conditions can bring immense disappointment. There has been the hope that the treatment had worked and/or that their prayers had been answered.

What follows are descriptions of some of the mindsets that patients may experience. According to your intuition and guidance there are many actions you could take or words you could say. Listen to their story. How are they relating to self, others, community, God? Your understanding of their emotional reactions will help you be more effective in your ministry approach.

The **most beneficial actions** are to:
> Radiate love.
> Offer your full attention—a listening presence—without
>   judgment.
> Show sensitivity and acceptance.
> Exude caring and compassion; empathize.
> Pray when appropriate.
> Read or quote scripture.
> Leave them an inspirational book.

Here are a few suggestions specific to various situations to get you started. As you think of more, add them to the list. Remember that you are not there to "fix". *The most powerful medicine is to be totally present and focused as if no one else existed in the world at that moment. Your time with the patient should be brief but profound.*

When you **pray**, focus on:

> Gratitude (for loved ones, staff, medical science, opportunities in this health crises, God's care and presence, whatever else you are aware of that you can praise God about.)
>
> Forgiveness for patient and others.
>
> Need for God's support/strength; His presence in the room during surgery or procedures.
>
> Trust in God. Trust God's will or destiny for patient.

Other things you might do to help, if you are trained:

> Relaxation methods, deep breathing
>
> Imagery or visualization
>
> Healing humor/laughter (If it won't hurt them physically.)
>
> Give them something tangible:
>
>> a card with a biblical quote to reflect on
>>
>> an encouraging word, stone or heart
>>
>> some momentum or object of importance to them

THE PATIENT'S DILEMMAS/POSSIBLE MIND SETS:

- **Anxiety**

    About seriousness, nature or duration of illness.

    Whether or not they will have to have an operation.

    Whether or not it is curable.

    Self talk: Will the doctor ever get here?

    Is it hereditary?

    Is it contagious?

    Will they tell me the truth?

    Do I want to know the truth?

    How am I going to live with this?

    (Ex. Amputation)

    How will I recover financially?

    Will I make a fool of myself?

    How much will it hurt? Can I take it?

    What can you do?

    You can't fix it, but you can offer encouragement:

    One day at a time. Right now we need you to
    focus on your recovery.

    We'll take the problems as they come.

    You can count on us to be here for you.

- **Ashamed**

    Of appearance

    Area of the body that is diseased or facing procedure

    Of tubes in and out

    To be toileted in bed

    Of being emotional

    Smell

<u>What can you do?</u>
Acknowledge the situation matter-of-factly (not pretending to notice or ignore it.)

<u>What not to do</u>
Show embarrassment.

- **Attention-Need of**
  Unhappy with life and world
  Need an excuse for not succeeding.
  Enjoy attention, protection, kindness, and care received in hospital.

  <u>What can you do?</u>
  Affirm their value.
  Attempt to involve them in church activities in some way.
  Instill a reason for living.

- **Cover-up**
  Jolly, putting on a happy face
  Don't want to talk about themselves, rather talk about you or the weather or....
  (This could be genuine or also signal a reluctance to deal with reality.)

  <u>What can you do?</u>
  Probe

- **Depressed**
  Little eye contact
  No vitality
  Sleep to escape or unable to sleep at all.

<u>What can you do?</u>

Get them talking about something that will remind them of a blessing.

Relate hopefulness in some form.

> Ex. If the room has flowers or cards, say, "My look at all the expressions of love in your room!" or "There are many of us praying for you and are here for you as you go through this health crises."(If that is true.)

- **Disoriented/Difficulty tracking or comprehending**

  Part of Dementia

  Reaction to strong medication

  <u>What can you do?</u>

  Be brief, simple.

- **Distrust of the medical system**

  Perception, real or imagined, feels like loss of control over their life.

  If procedures haven't been fully or properly explained

  Hatred of taking drugs

  Perception of being experimented on—Guinea pig affect

  <u>Self talk:</u> Will the doctor ever get here?

  > Will they tell me the truth?

  > Will I be in pain?

  <u>What can you do?</u>

  Encourage or precipitate a patient/doctor consult.

  Suggest a Bio-ethics consult if appropriate.

- **Emotions near the surface**

    Might be fear, sense of abandonment

    Unresolved issues with loved ones, may be expressed by:

    > Desire to resolve or reconcile
    >
    > Brooding or festering of emotions
    >
    > Explosive feelings

    <u>What can you do?</u>

    Reassure, encourage them to talk or cry.

    Encourage action when appropriate, such as call family members, forgive, reconcile.

    Help facilitate meeting, advocate for patient.

- **Fearful**

    Loss of control over one's environment causes stress, often expressed as fear.

    Procedures—Unclear about what exactly is being done (even if the procedure has been thoroughly explained and all questions answered).

    Wonder whether medical staff can be trusted.

    <u>Self talk:</u> Will I be able to understand what the medical staff is explaining?

    > What happens if it goes wrong?
    >
    > What if they find something else?
    >
    > How severe is this really?
    >
    > Will I ever be strong and healthy again?
    >
    > Will I be able to resume my work?
    >
    > Is something terrible going to happen to me?
    >
    > Am I ready to die?

<u>What can you do?</u>

Offer to pray before procedure or surgery begins.

Assure them that you will remain in prayer for them during scheduled procedure.

If possible, stay nearby and support family.

- **Guilt**

    For not protecting one's family (financial concerns, children "farmed out")

    For being sick in the first place (caused by poor self care, i.e. eating and sleep habits, over-working, smoking, drugs, drinking, etc.)

    About things said and unsaid to loved ones.

    Review of past sins, disobediences.

    <u>Self talk:</u> Why did this happen to me?

    Is it my fault?

    Is God punishing me?

    I waited too long.

    <u>What can you do?</u>

    Encourage forgiveness of self.

    Remind them that they can make changes in life-style and relationship investments.

- **Hopelessness/Helplessness/Loss of Freedom**

    Strange bed, strange place, strange people, strange odors

    Clothes removed, cannot come and go when they want to

    Bathroom-shared or unable to go alone, bedpan

    Loss of privacy

    Dietary changes or food different than used to

    Loss of control. Under someone else's agenda or orders, examinations, tests

    Depersonalization

<u>Self talk:</u> Where is the doctor? Nurse?

I can't manage this myself.

Nothing can help me—it's hopeless.

I never felt this way before.

<u>What can you do?</u>

Be patient, reassuring.

Talk positive about the hospital and medical team, if you can.

Ask where they have found hope in the past. Who inspired them?

- **Impatient/Irritable**

  Especially difficult for the elderly, hard of hearing, or those set in their ways with little flexibility.

  <u>Self talk:</u> I need help now.

  I feel stuck. Nothing I do is helpful.

  <u>What can you do?</u>

  Be patient, reassuring.

- **Indifference**

  Often a coping mechanism

  <u>What can you do?</u>

  Don't give up, persist.

- **Lonely or abandoned**

  By loved ones, friends, church community or God

  Homesickness

  Worry about family while away

  Children easily fall into this category, often exhibiting separation anxiety from their parents.

  <u>Self talk:</u> Can they get along without me? Suppose they learn they can?

  Are they glad/relieved I'm not there?

  Perhaps they will forget me! Not want me back! Find someone else!

  <u>What can you do?</u>

  Hug appropriately if you have permission.

  Notify friends or family to support.

  <u>What not to do</u>

  Defend God or preach

- **Loss of dignity**

  Hospital gown-size and openness

  Embarrassing procedures

  Restrained from bathroom privileges

  <u>What can you do?</u>

  Knock before entering and ask if you can come in.

  Always leave if a nurse or doctor arrives.

- **Loss of privacy**

   Door to their temporary bedroom is open to public view.

   Roommate, (staff, visitors, family) are coming and going.

   <u>What can you do?</u>

   Knock before entering and ask if you can come in.

   Always leave if a nurse or doctor arrives.

- **Sleep deprived**

   Circadian rhythm disturbed.

   Noises in general (roommate snoring or having TV on, cleaners, staff)

   Awakened to receive medication or vitals taken

   <u>Self talk:</u> I can't think clearly. I'm going crazy.

   My mind isn't working right.

   <u>What can you do?</u>

   Let sleeping patient sleep.

   Tip toe in and leave your card or give to patient's nurse.

- **Sufferng/Pain**

   Can cause fear

   Can cause mood swings, irritability, hopelessness.

   Can become self-focused and often cannot relate to others as they'd like to.

   <u>Self talk:</u> Will they give me something for the pain?

   Should I take it? Will I get addicted?

   Will I become handicapped or deformed?

   Will I become an invalid and have to be waited on or cared for?

   What about my job?

<u>What can you do?</u>

Make empathetic remarks such as:

> "I realize that with all this suffering you're not yourself."

> "I'm so sorry you're in pain."

- **Unable to follow religious practices that bring comfort**

<u>What can you do?</u>

Discuss needs with hospital chaplain or nurse. Hospital standards require opportunities to meet spiritual needs of the patient.

- **Why me?**

It isn't fair.

God has forsaken me, abandon me, is punishing me, doesn't love me.

This is because of what I did…

<u>What can you do?</u>

Say something like: "His shoulders are big enough for your questions, or anger. Just don't get stuck there. Life isn't fair. It's not necessary to pull away from God."

- **Worthlessness**

When not able to fulfill an accustomed role, such as bread winner

<u>What can you do?</u>

Encourage them that things have a way of working out.

Remind them God's hand is over them and has promised provision.

The bottom line is to put yourself in the patient's place and consider their discomfort, fears and needs. Look into the depths of their eyes and listen beyond their words to their heart. Allow God to be His hands, words, and love through you; then you will experience the miraculous. Your visit will be successful and appreciated.

SUMMARY: WHAT PATIENT'S WANT/NEED

- For you to ask how they are doing spiritually.
- Listen without judgment.
- Keep confidentialities.
- Take their concerns seriously.
- Be truthful.
- Convey hope or offer encouragement of God's grace, mercy, comfort, strength.
- Help them make their own decisions.
- Help them focus on their quality of life not length.
- Keep your focus on companionship, comfort, conversaation, and consultation.
- Spend time with them as needed and as they can tolerate.
- Reassure them of your love and concern, and God's.

SUMMARY: BARRIERS TO SPIRITUAL CARE

- Guilt, sense of not feeling worthy, resistant, loss of self-esteem.
- Has a hidden story.
- No strength to self-help.
- Anxiety levels continually changing due to medical awareness and care.

- Inability to process health/diagnostic information.
- Fear
- Lack of self-discipline to carry out medical orders.
- Forgiveness issues.
- Have not been attending church. Lack of interest or angry at God.
- Conflict over lack of commitment to Christ/church prior to medical crises.
- Unable to pray or read Bible. (Too hard to understand.)
- Relying on others' beliefs, opinions, advice, or feelings.

Pastoral Tools

Pastoral conversation is the primary tool in relationship. So the minister in order to be effective must be a skilled communicator. This means more than the ability to verbalize. It includes the fine art of **listening** without showing shock or dismay at what we see or hear. *(See Chapter—Visitation Etiquette, Section: Caring Communication)*

Our personality is what impacts the individual and the situation. We should have an awareness of our relational pattern and the way we communicate both verbally and nonverbally. Dr. G. Howard Litton states, "The real self of the pastor in relationship, is personality." He recognizes the minister's role as the most significant contributing factor of effectiveness in the care of the sick and presents a number of "tools of the trade" as effective resources in ministry.

PASTORAL RESOURCES:

In this chapter we will include a number of tools, with an explanation of appropriate usage. Spiritual gifts may be needed more than flowers, candy, balloons, or stuffed animals.
We will discuss the use of:

      Anointing
      Prayer/Claiming Bible Promises
      Baby Dedication
      Rituals/Relaxation Response

Baptism
Sacred Symbols of Sacraments/Ordinances
Healing Baskets/Supportive Actions
Music/Singing/Praise/Hymns
Scripture/Encouraging Readings

Hospitals respect the ecumenical nature of their patient population and are generally most accommodating when this is communicated to them. Do not hesitate in inviting the staffs' participation when they are available.

If there is another patient in the room, provision needs to be made so there is no detrimental effect on them when ministering to the needs of your parishioner. Give the staff the opportunity to make room changes or provide privacy when you are administering communion, dedications, baptisms, anointing with oil, laying on of hands; especially if there is to be a loud service such as speaking in tongues or deliverance counseling.

ANOINTING

In James 5:14 we are admonished to call the elders, anoint with oil and make confession. It is assumed that those involved in the anointing service will have been encouraged to spend time with God in advance, doing some heart searching and preparation; making sure that all is well between them and God and all sins are confessed.

Oil, which has been consecrated to God's service, should be used. Some anoint by marking a spot of oil on the forehead, others make a cross with the oil on the forehead. Generally both ways are accompanied with the words," I now anoint you in the name of the Father, the Son, and the Holy Spirit (Ghost).

Put some thought into this sacred time. Following your tradition, be sure and make the anointing service special. You could sing some songs, read some scripture, or share a testimony. Each person participating can pray, or you alone can bless the patient. Be creative.

BABY DEDICATION

Ask staff when a convenient time is and invite their attendance and or participation. Words of love and blessing should be summoned from God. He knows what His destiny for this child is and will gladly anoint your lips. A good resource to use during dedication is the "Name Book" by Dorothy Astoria (ISBN 1-55661-982-0) which gives the spiritual meanings of baby's name. After reading the definition, prayer could be offered. Ask God's protection over the child. Ask that (s)he will live to fulfill the meaning of her/his name. Baby Dedication Certificates are sometimes available at the Chaplain/Spiritual Care Department.

BAPTISM

It is rarely possible to do a baptism by immersion in the hospital unless the patient is mobile enough. In that event, unless death is forthcoming, it would be prudent to conduct baptism after the patient is released. If death is forthcoming, it is advisable to come up with an alternative plan, such as pouring water over the feet—similar to a foot washing service— symbolic of baptism, on the forehead, or anointing with oil--a symbol of spiritual healing.

HEALING BASKETS AND SUPPORTIVE ACTIONS

Family members that spend a considerable time in the hospital room with a failing or recovering patient often neglect their own needs. A basket of healthy snacks, encouraging notes, suitable reading material, games, books, and toiletries is another way of saying, "We care." Include items that the patient might need as well.

Family members are pulled in many directions, just to keep up with life, as they stand by the patient. Church members can convey messages, send food, help care for other children, clean the house and prepare it for the patient's return. All of this should be done with permission as to not embarrass or offend the family.

MUSIC/SINGING—PRAISE AND HYMNS

Music is wonderfully soothing, encouraging and healing. Whether the music is instrumental or vocal, whether spiritually produced in familiar hymns or contemporary praise, it can be uplifting and change the attitude and perspective of the patients as they become absorbed in it. It can be as effective to the unconscious patient as well, and give them reason to hold on to life or peacefully surrender to God's plan. Use music respectfully if the patient has a roommate.

PRAYER/CLAIMING BIBLE PROMISES

Prayer should be offered after you have had a meaningful interaction with the person, and have explored areas of concern and importance. In a crisis situation, prayer, readings, or claiming Scripture promises, can be calming; emphasizing the resources of peace, strength, courage, quietness, fellowship and hope. It is also healing to hold hands when praying. With many Christian groups, comfort is found in repeating the Lord's Prayer together. Form a prayer circle around the bed with family, holding hands to bring unity to the attendees.

Misuse:
Prayer can be used in a way of providing the simple solution to a complex problem--shifting all responsibility to God instead of allowing the patient to investigate their need to make lifestyle adjustments. Unfortunately, some ministers are tempted to use prayer to preach something that they feel unable to address directly. This is inappropriate. Prayer is also used to help make a graceful exit because there is a sense that it is expected. Don't feel you <u>have to</u> pray. Follow the leading of the Holy Spirit.

Positive implications:
Prayer should present to God the feelings and perspectives of the patient, without judgment. It should make a place for negative feelings. Prayer can release buried emotions so healing can take place. Prayer, shared with discernment, can assist in giving reinforcement for the "will to live" and help break the cycle of pain, bringing comfort and strength. *(See chapter on Healing Scriptures and Prayers.)*

Applying Scripture as we pray, incorporating the healing, protective, caring promises of God, is one of the greatest gifts towards peace. Submitting the patient's future for God to fulfill His destiny in their life, can bring them calm and peace, not of this world.

Suggested application:
To work together with God for healing or comfort, one should begin their prayers with praise. In offering the Prayer of Faith, we see that Scripture teaches that praise dispels the enemy and gives us access to heaven. God inhabits the praises of His people. Next we are to offer confessions and ask for forgiveness. (James 5:16, 1John 1:9) Now present your intercession, your supplications before God, (Matthew 7:7,8) thanking Him in advance for His answers (Philippians 4:6). As you pray, mention scriptural promises, reminding God of what He has done in the past. *(See chapter on Healing Promises.)*

RITUALS/RELAXATION RESPONSE

The familiarity of sacred rituals can bring much peace to the patient. Sharing a meaningful and known prayer together, or other traditions of your faith, has the ability of decreasing the patient's blood pressure and reducing an elevated heart rate. Dr. Herbert Benson ascertains that the relaxation response provides a direct linkage to faith in something beyond.

SACRED SYMBOLS OF SACRAMENTS/ORDINANCES

Sacraments/Ordinances are acts which have meanings deeper than words, because of what they symbolize and the longtime traditions attached to them. The mystical effect of communion, also referred to as the Eucharist, identifies with Christ and the church. For the very spiritual/religious patient, the sacraments or spiritual symbols can symbolize their eternal future/destiny and is of significant importance that they be administered; particularly to the Catholic patient.

The grape juice/wine symbolizes Christ's sacrifice and cleansing blood, which offers forgiveness of sins and new beginnings. The bread/wafer, which symbolizes Christ's body, offers healing according to the text in Isaiah 54:4-5 which proclaims that the Lord "took up our infirmities, carried our sorrows and by his stripes we are healed".

Communion may require permission from the doctor or nurse to be sure the patient can ingest the elements. Communicating with staff regarding the time you will be administrating sacraments, will provide needed privacy, which generally is respected, or an inclusion of staff members as appropriate. For the sacraments to be of greatest value to the patient, the minister must understand what they mean to the person at this time, in this specific experience. If the patient is unable to have the communion bread, you might ask the hospital chaplain if meltable wafers are available to place in the juice/wine.

SCRIPTURE/ENCOURAGING READINGS
Scripture can hinder or help

Hindrance:
The timing, when ministering with scripture, can be critical to the healing and hope for the patient's eternal future. This is not a time for condemnation, but for encouragement and salvation. Using scripture before the patient has had an opportunity to explore the depth of their concerns, may be premature. This is especially so if they are intensely and totally absorbed in personal conflicts such as: pain, fear, resentment, hostility, grief, anger or situational stress. When the time comes to use scripture, if a pa-

tient is struggling with their feelings toward God, or is angry with Him, then a more generic reading might be more effective to begin with.

Help

When using scripture as a point of identification, for a source of courage and strength, or for comfort, it can help the patient be conscious of God's awareness of their situation. It can also be a diagnostic tool to help you become aware of the deeper heart issues that need addressing. You can instruct, inform, teach, and comfort. Depending on the emotional and spiritual health and current perspective of the patient, it might be more advisable to read an encouraging thought that will give them the comfort, hope, courage and reminder that God is with them. Biblical promises can be incorporated when they are more open to hearing them. *(See chapter on Healing Scriptures and Prayers.)*

Story: I visited a Korean War veteran that was riddled with guilt for killing a young "enemy". He said, "I haven't slept through the night since then. I can't go on like this. I have been to counseling. I have prayed. I went to a priest. He said, "Go and sin no more." Nothing has helped me.

I was deep in prayer as to how to minister to this man. God gave me 1 John 1:9, "If we confess our sins, He is faithful and just to forgive us our sins and cleanse us from all unrighteousness." Then God prompted me to say, "Maybe you need to ask God to forgive you for not believing Him."

We prayed. I claimed that promise for him. At the close of our prayer, his countenance had changed. He glowed. He was smiling from ear to ear. He said, "Something has happened to me. I have never felt this way before."

That night he slept through the night. God healed him. Though he had been told that he would be in the hospital for four to five days, he was discharged the next morning.

Ministering to Various Populations

As ministers, we represent to a patient God's presence, the love of God, His healing power, and community support. Our presence can also precipitate a sense of guilt and a need to confess. In light of this, there is a need to emphasize to the patient the truth of God's word, "If we confess our sins, He is faithful and just to forgive us our sins and cleanse us from all unrighteousness." (1 John 1:9) Also, "A cheerful heart doeth good like medicine." (Proverbs 17:22)

In the medical field, there is a growing recognition that any breakdown of health in any area; physical, mental or spiritual, effects the overall health in the other areas. For example, many people are hospitalized because they have been carrying unforgiveness. Either they have not forgiven others, self, or God. Commonly, when life does not play out the way anticipated, and trials and heartache interrupt, people get angry with God. After all, they are "good" people and try to live a virtuous life. Why would God allow such heartache in their life? When they choose not to forgive, they become judgmental, critical, resentful, angry, depressed, discouraged, etc. This causes stress, which breaks down their body forces and sets them up for disease. Consequently, one of the major issues to be addressed is whether or not our patient is reconciled on all levels.

Many times I have asked a patient if everything is right between them and others, and them and God. Often they have replied, "Yes, it is." I have asked, "No unfinished business? No unsettled issues where forgiveness is needed?" They have said something like, "No, everything is fine. I've taken care of everything." Then I have responded with, "What about you? Have you forgiven yourself?" Nine times out of ten they begin to cry. Now we were able to make progress! Healing could begin.

I ask them, "Are you ready to forgive yourself or do you want to carry this around a little longer and make sure you've sufficiently punished yourself?" I usually get a look of surprise or questioning eyebrows. I repeat with a smile, "Are you ready to forgive yourself so that you can leave the hospital with all of your "baggage" left behind and go home with new beginnings?" 99% of the time this ends up in further discussion and a deep healing experience.

It is important to note, ***"healing is not always cure"***. God's greatest concern is the healing of our hearts that are assured of our salvation and reconciled to Him.

Our ministry will be most effective if we remember that all people have an innate drive to:
- understand what is happening to them and why
- be aware of what gives meaning to who they are and what they do
- (This could be God, their family, or position)
- change whatever is causing unhappiness or pain in their life
- hang on to hope no matter what the crises

The spiritual piece of each of us reaches out for faith, hope, love, for a sense of meaning and purpose for our life, for a reason to live, and an understanding of the events we are currently facing.

Our unique role is to assess with the patient such issues as:
- What is of prime importance in their belief/value system?
- How can the patient be empowered to hope/cope and draw strength from their relationship to God here and now? Is it possible to be sad and disappointed and still find things to be thankful for and laugh about? Yes!
- How has the patient found the strength to cope with negative experiences in the past?
- What brings joy and peace into their life?
- What sources do they have for a support team during this difficult time? Are they estranged from their support system?
- Are they realistic about their present situation?

We can understand that when patients are hospitalized, they:
- may have separation anxiety from family or friends.
- may have concerns about the welfare of their family.
- may have feelings of helplessness, a loss of freedom, and/or depression.
- may have a fear of the unknown and the strangeness of the hospital; wondering whether or not the hospital staff can be trusted.
- may fear the inability to deal with their pain or the inability to cope with the illness or disability.
- may have anxiety about their illness and of being a burden to caregivers or becoming dependent on others. An independent person fights being dependent on anyone.

- may have a variety of fears: of pain, handicap, loss of mobility, deformity, whether they will be an invalid for life, and how others will respond to and accept them.
- may wonder if their family misses them or if they are glad they are away.
- are experiencing concern about their job.
- are worried about finances.
- may be struggling with a sense of guilt or unresolved issues of forgiveness.
- could feel a threat of surgery or death and a concern as to whether or not they are ready.
- may have unfinished business.

Illness and incapacitation is not an individual matter. Every person that the patient's life touches can be affected. Be sensitive to what family members or caretakers are going through; the pressure they are under, the fatigue of having to assume additional responsibilities or care and their need of support and understanding. Ask the caregiver how they're doing. Family and caregivers are as much a part of your ministry outreach as is the patient. Often they are more in need of support than the patient.

When we know that one of our parishioners is in the hospital, the tendency is to work a visit into our already packed schedule. Seldom do we stop to realize that our ministry will be different according to sex, age, or situation of the person we hope to touch. Included in this chapter will be numerous approaches to use under varying circumstances. Your innate discernment and guidance from the Holy Spirit will help you know which ones are applicable to the situation you are ministering in. Not all will be used, and the succession is variable.

In this chapter you will discover ways to minister to:

Young Adults/Adults	Surgery Patients
Children	Intensive Care and
	Emergency Room Patients
To Parents	Comatose
Adolescent	Chronically Ill
Elderly	Serious Illness
Disabled	Critically or Terminally Ill
Blind	Dying and Bereaved

Keep in mind that one of your most valuable resources is the hospital Chaplain who can guide your visit based upon information they have gathered during rounds.

MINISTERING TO YOUNG ADULTS/ADULTS

Note that it is often easier for women to express their feelings and for men to ignore or stuff their feelings. Encourage open sharing by asking thoughtful, probing, but appropriate questions, and clarifying what you hear.

- Recognize that their focus is on family, career, earning power, financial security.
- Establish rapport by finding common interests.
- Ask them for their perception of the situation.
- Try to see things from their perspective.
- Avoid asking a lot of questions. Let them volunteer. Patients tire of repeating story.
- Establish that you are a "safe place" for them to share their struggles and questions.
- Encourage expression of feelings, thoughts, and behaviors.
- Affirm patient's experiences, their pain and their courage in seeking help.

- Help them understand their identity from a biblical perspective.
- Be sensitive to the fact that many men are more visual than auditory or feeling-centered and women are more sensitive, relational and feeling centered.
- Help them focus on immediate needs and resources rather than on seeking approval.
- Avoid caretaking behaviors that may delay the acceptance of their condition, behaviors and responsibilities.
- Show patient through words and actions that you have faith in their ability to manage their life and to set goals for continued progress.
- Determine their level of spiritual development and help work out a plan for spiritual growth which will reflect their strengths and needs.
- Ask the patient to highlight their God-given abilities, strengths, spiritual gifts and capabilities. If they struggle, assist patient in identifying them.
- Challenge patient to work toward maturity in Christ, integrating emotional, intellectual, social and spirit wholeness; especially during the time of crises.
- Note spiritual concerns or distress. These could include discouragement, anticipatory grief, inability to participate in usual religious practices, concern about their relationship with God, struggle with guilt. Any anger at staff, family, or God, may interrupt their spiritual trust, and cause them to feel distant from God at a time when they need Him most. They may become increasingly concerned about their relationship with God as their illness progresses.

- Invite them to share their story. Much of a person's spirituality is contained in their story. As they share, identify their source of spiritual strength in coping with past crisis or illness.
- Share your faith, stories. Leave them with a sense of hope.

MINISTERING TO CHILDREN

Often illness and hospitalization are the first crises children must face. Their reaction to these crises is influenced by developmental age, previous experience with illness, separation, acquired coping skills, the seriousness of the diagnosis and the support system available. The child patient challenges everyone to work together to offer the child understanding, compassion, security, love, faith, and hope. The minister's assistance may be most significant in assisting the parents.

A common question from a parent is:
How much should the child know about their diagnosis and prognoses? A sense of foreboding and distrust can arise in the child if they perceive there are secrets. Usually, the medical staff is in agreement that including the child with their parents in the communication, is the most desirable.

Common family crisis problems when a child is suffering/hospitalized:
Healthcare crises can strengthen or weaken family relationships. Marital conflict can emerge. Parents can play the blame game. If it is an injury, "Why wasn't the child being watched?" If it is genetic, "It's your side." Parents can also absorb the guilt, sometimes believing and accepting that this is a punishment for something they have done or said.

They might also ascribe the blame to God. This can result in alienation from God as well as self-alienation precipitating communication problems—difficulty talking about it. All of this can create conflict between the parents as they may have different perspectives regarding the care of the child, outcome, hope and future, or religious beliefs/spiritual practices.

Parents or adult family members may be overtired and stressed from taking turns staying at the hospital and being separated from each other. They may have difficulty keeping up with things at home or work, or are concerned about other children. Other children may become problematic if they feel they are being neglected, have thoughts that there is favoritism or feel in any way that this is their fault.

Primary parent staying with the patient-child becomes communication link between hospital (the doctors and staff) and spouse and family. The parent, not in the immediate loop can feel disintegrated and often protect themselves by emotional distancing.

Sexual inactivity and intimacy may suffer if one or both feel guilt or fear of producing another imperfect or ill child. Another form of guilt is manifested during a long term illness when a family member might wish the child would die. They feel unable to cope any longer and don't want their child to suffer or continue in the present state.

Hard times bring out our insecurities. "What did I do to deserve this?" "Doesn't anyone care?" "Where is everyone?" "I don't matter." "God has abandoned me."

INFANTS:

- Be aware that infants mimic.
- Smile and use facial expressions of happiness.
- Repeat actions that elicit response; waving, peek-a-boo, pat-a-cake
- Model desired behavior.
- Build trust.
- Ask parent's permission to touch patient. Touch should be gentle and loving.

TODDLERS:

- Recognize that they are too young to use reason and are often impatient with a short attention span.
- Know that imagination and reality are the same to them.
- They are attached to security objects and toys.
- Realize that a toddler may respond with physical aggression and be verbally uncooperative.
- Exude gentleness and patience with a peaceful and loving countenance.
- Tell the child it is okay to cry.
- Use distraction techniques.
- Use few and simple terms that are familiar to the child.
- Use play; simple games or read to them.
- Allow choices whenever possible.
- They enjoy religious rituals such as prayer before meals and bedtime. Invite them to pray with you.

SCHOOL AGE:

- Recognize that they are generally striving for approval but may passively withdraw.
- Encourage self expression.
- Compliment the child on his/her accomplishments.
- Encourage the child to verbalize ideas and feelings.
- Know that they are able to handle and classify problems.
- Understand that they function in the present.
- Acknowledge that you understand that they prefer their friends to family and that gaining approval from their peer group is important to them.
- Inquire about their accomplishments at school. They are proud of this.
- Praise child for helping and cooperating.
- Relate to their abilities and dreams.
- Suggest ways of maintaining control.
- Play games with rules.
- Address their fear of "loss of control".
- Address their need to know that God has not abandoned them and that they are not being punished for wrong thoughts or behaviors. They have the spiritual need for forgiveness and freedom of guilt. They believe in good and evil and spend time thinking about what God does and how He does it. Help them deal with feelings of anger towards God.

ADOLESCENT:

- Recognize their struggles for independence, self assertion and seeking for personal identity. They are sometimes angry about the need to conform.
- Be mindful that privacy is of utmost importance to these patients. Show respect.
- Respect their fear of physical exposure. They are focused on their physical appearance.
- Realize that they may fear death, disability or other potential risks.
- Encourage questions regarding fears, options and alternatives.
- Help them realize the significance of the immediate effects of the procedure they are facing or have been through. They may be concerned if they have taken on additional responsibilities such as jobs and leadership roles at school.
- Suggest methods of maintaining control.
- Speak to them as though they were an adult.
- Speak to them with recognition that they are capable of developing a deep relationship with God. They have a need for meaning, purpose and hope in life and are asking "Who am I?" They are wondering why there is suffering. They are in need of the reassurance that God is in control and can support them through this crisis.
- Model God's care and love showing that you are concerned about the patient and that they are valued.
- Treat their confusion with compassion respecting their dignity.

MNISTERING TO THE PARENTS:

- Addressing issues in advance can protect and enrich marriage by helping them affirm their love as parents and also affirming God's love.
- Help coordinate parent's visitation if they are divorced and there is tension between them.
- Assist and/or encourage parents to go through a time of reflection and reprioritize life demands and involvements.
- Advise parents that when they are tearful around their hospitalized child, to let their child know: "Mommy doesn't like to see you hurting" (or not feeling well). "It's okay for me to let my feelings out just like you do when you're unhappy." This frees up child to be honest about their feelings.
- Remember to visit with and support siblings. Turn this into an opportunity to build trust, enhance relationships and validate your interest in and concern for each family member—offsetting jealousy and self-condemnation.
- Promptly enlist help from church members, particularly for single parents. (Members that are understanding and nonjudgmental.)
- Encourage open communication and support. Terminally ill children are sometimes feared to be contagious and can be abandoned by playmates. Family is often not included in social functions. They will hear excuses such as "We didn't want to disturb or bother you."
- Arrange a date with the child patient. Visit at a time when you can relieve the parents to have time together or go for a meal. Bring a game to play with the child, a book to read or watch TV together. Puppets are very helpful and can encourage a child to share feelings.

- Remember children have the same feelings as adults do—fear, anger, loneliness, guilt, sadness, hope, anticipation, the need to trust, to love and know they are loved—not abandoned.
- Pray mentioning how Jesus loves children and that nothing can separate us from His love.

MINISTERING TO ELDERLY

Six criteria of well-being in old age as determined by Carol Ryff, are self-acceptance, positive relations with others, autonomy (personal freedom), environmental mastery, purpose for life and continued personal growth. Focus on these factors as you interact with this population.

- Wear bright and warm colors
- Comment on the day, season, and local news in a natural way to help keep isolated persons in touch with reality.
- Allow silences to give patient time to say what he wants. Sitting in silence can be surprisingly companionable.
- Inquire and listen to their underlying feelings and tell them what you think they said.
- Listen carefully to complaints and ask them what they can do about their complaint.

- Listen for acceptance of what has been and for their present journey.
- Beware of any clue towards loneliness, bitterness, or atrophy.
- Gently challenge a patient that is being "too nice" with "You can be honest with me."
- Listen to fantasies, visions or hallucinations. Admit they sound strange to you. If applicable, check the story with staff.

- Ask for more details and introduce a new idea or item of interest if they tell you something over and over.
- Tell a patient in pain that you wish you could help, but you can't; but you would like to be with him. Exhibit appropriate touching or holding and crying with them.
- Key yourself to patient's mood and position.
- Discuss their decision, but do not make it for them, when they ask you what they should do.
- Show appropriate affection.
- Question them to see if they have an acceptable understanding of life after death. Note if they have given up or are still involved in things that bring meaning to their life.
- Remind them that they are a valuable source of skill, knowledge and lessons from life experiences.
- Note spiritual concerns or distress. These could include discouragement, anticipatory grief, inability to participate in usual religious practices, concern about their relationship with God, struggle with guilt. Any anger at staff, family, or God, may interrupt their spiritual trust, and cause them to feel distant from God at a time when they need Him most. They become increasingly concerned about their relationship with God as their illness progresses.
- Invite them to share their story. Much of a person's spirituality is contained in their story. As they share, identify their source of spiritual strength in coping with past crisis or illness.
- Share your faith, stories of faith, prayers, read aloud. Leave them with a sense of hope.
- Make only promises you can keep when scheduling a revisit.

MINISTERING TO DISABLED PATIENTS

- Show respect and encouragement. Be natural. Remember they are not incapable they just have limitations due to their handicap.
- Don't pretend that the disability doesn't exist. Show interest in them.
- Build friendship and trust. Encourage them to share their heart concerns and adjustment challenges.
- Be courteous. Don't scrutinize everything they do.
- Laugh. Be yourself. Let your conversation flow freely and comfortably.
- Assist patient only when they request it; or offer and wait for a response. Being too helpful or overly protective can be offensive and embarrassing.
- Allow the patient to set their own pace when walking or "wheeling around."
- Separating them from their wheelchair or crutches should only be done after consulting them. Keep the apparatus nearby to help them feel more secure.
- Assist them with cutting food at mealtime if they are in need of help.
- Share appropriate scriptures and pray. In many cases, you may be surprised at how inspired you will be after your visit. Their determination and good humor will be refreshing.

MINISTERING TO BLIND PATIENTS

- Show respect and encouragement. Be natural. Remember they are not incapable; they just can't see.
- Announce yourself when entering the room.

- Speak directly in a normal conversational tone.
- Guide the patient by inviting them to take your arm. Move forward at your regular pace, slightly ahead of them, but conscious of their ability to move at that pace.
- Give directions specifically, such as "right" or "left".
- Always let them know if you are coming to a curb, stairs, or uneven ground.
- Describe the surroundings when in public.
- Seat the patient by placing their hand on the arm of the back of the chair and by allowing them to seat themselves.
- Instruct them, when eating, on location of food using cues like the numbers on a clock: such as "salad at 9:00 o'clock, potatoes at 6:00 o'clock, etc.
- Assist them during entrance to vehicle. Place one hand on the door handle and one on top of the car. Tell them which direction the vehicle is facing.

MINISTERING TO SURGERY PATIENTS

According to one doctor, if you think the surgery is minor, consider that any time the surgeon picks up the knife, and the anesthesiologist is called, it is serious. Families need comforting. Sometimes they are terrified. If the doctor says surgery will take an hour or two, and then it goes on for three or four hours, their imagination can go wild. If you can't stay the whole time, check back by phone or in person with the family to help them through this.

- Be sure you are aware of patient's surgery time and how early you can come.
- Key yourself to patient's mood and emotional mind set.
- Be sensitive to family and support needed.

- Articulate faith in staff. "I've heard good things about the staff here."
- Pray—*(See section on Prayers)*

MINISTERING TO PATIENTS IN INTENSIVE CARE AND EMERGENCY ROOM: This may include victims of accidents, violence, or abuse.

- Check with the nurse before seeing the patient.
- Make your visit extremely brief when in ICU. In ER you may be needed to hold hands and divert their attention.
- Communicate by touch—gently on the shoulder or by squeezing the patient's hand when (s)he is on a ventilator.
- Encourage uplifting communication and words of hope, if appropriate, around the bedside of a person in a coma. They often hear what is being said.
- Be sensitive to needs of family and offer support.
- Encourage family and speak words of hope if appropriate.
- Determine, to the best of your ability, the depth of spirituality of the patient and the spirituality and tradition of family members or caretakers you are also ministering to.
- Assist reconciling any unresolved issues between family and patient.
- Pray intercession and forgiveness when appropriate.
- Pray for them to envision Jesus at the foot of their bed with His arms of love open to them.

MINISTRY TO THE COMATOSE PATIENT

- The last of the five senses to stop functioning are touch (pads of hand and fingers), and hearing. Even when you don't think the patient can hear you, they can be acutely aware. Positive dialogue by the bedside is crucial.
- Make sure that the conversations around the bedside are affirming, encouraging, hopeful, and positive. Do not allow any negative or "terminal" conversations within patient's hearing.
- Identify yourself and acknowledge that you understand they are unable to speak.
- Let them know that you came to be with them.
- You want them to know that you, their family, church family and God cares.
- Reassure them that you are all praying for them.
- Invite them to squeeze your hand if they understand. (Don't be concerned if they don't)
- Read scripture, pray, sing, anoint with oil (if appropriate).

MINISTERING TO THE CHRONICALLY ILL

This is generally a long illness requiring convalescence and life changes.

- Ascertain whether or not patient is lonely; they often have a lot of spare time on their hands. Since they are not in a critical condition, they do not receive constant care. If they are home bound, caretakers might lose their sensitivity to patient's needs.
- Question to find out if the patient has accepted their condition or is brooding, fallen into self-pity, or has too

much spare time. Come up with constructive activities/
church involvement. Help them feel useful and needed.
Do not reward self-pity but anticipate that they will have
hard times occasionally; be supportive.

- Exude genuine understanding of condition and feelings.
If they are handicapped, they may exhibit frustration, resentment, or hostilities and decide not to put the energy
into healing or improving their condition.
- Avoid being offended personally if aggression or hostilities are expressed. Offer hope. Do not discuss this behavior with others that will visit. Let them identify it.
- Give companionship...personally. Interest others to visit
the patient. Give suggestions as to how they can support
and encourage patient.
- Provide appropriate devotional and spiritually uplifting
reading material or taped sermons.
- Provide copies of the sermon and sacraments if they are
not able to attend church.
- Recognize their personal value. Their self-esteem can be
destroyed if you are patronizing or condescending.

MINISTRY TO THE PATIENT WITH A SERIOUS ILLNESS

- Keep your friendship strong. This is not the time to ne-
glect it.
- Send a card to let patient know you are thinking of them.
- Call before visiting; make sure it is an okay time.
- Tell the patient what you would like to do for them and
wait for agreement.
- Ask the patient if they feel like talking about what they
are going through, facing?

- Weep, laugh, share. Be sensitive to patient's needs/moods.
- Touch them. A gentle squeeze or handshake.
- Sit quietly if the patient isn't feeling communicative or is too ill.
- Bring a positive presence, peaceful spirit, hopeful perspective.
- Bring over a favorite meal in disposable containers.
- Bring music, posters, inspirational flip cards or books.
- Bring cookies for the family.
- Offer transportation to appointments or for children as needed.
- Help the family. Offer to sit with patient and give family a break/time out.
- Help with laundry, washing dishes, or housecleaning.
- Water flowers.
- Pray with the patient and family around bedside and share your faith.

MINISTERING TO THE CRITICALLY OR TERMINALLY ILL

This patient is generally facing a health crisis with a threat of death. Condition could improve or deteriorate. It encompasses attitude as well as prognosis.

- Try to find out patient's condition from medical staff. Patient may think they are in critically condition when is no immediate danger.
- Find patient's emotional level and minister at that point. Are they coping or succumbing? They may be severely depressed or overly optimistic. Don't avoid them. Their

first struggle is to deal with shock and still make wise decisions re: treatments, alternatives, doctors, etc.

- Remember in their mind, patient may feel they are losing control. Respect their personal limits/boundaries. The patient may be annoyed by the attitude of the medical staff. The patient might think of them as too calm or too casual.
- Determine the patient's desires. Patient may want visitors constantly or prefer to be alone. Patient may want to talk about their condition or avoid any discussion about it.
- Be aware of patient's current condition. Patient may feel severe pain or have none at all. Don't take offense if they are "short" with you or out of sorts. The question they may be asking in their mind but not verbalizing in their anger is: "How could you understand how I feel? You've never been through it."
- Bring a calm, composed and relaxed spirit into the room. This will help them develop faith—in you, themselves, staff, situation, and God.
- Watch your own feelings and reactions. Do not be upset or nervous.
- Bring a positive attitude. Talk about the future. Bring hope. How do the patient and family define hope?
- Don't feel you always have to talk. Sometimes just sitting silently and being present is most meaningful.
- Help patient feel good/comfortable about their appearance, considering their illness.
- Water their flowers for them.
- Give them an opportunity to talk about their feelings. Ask, "Do you feel like talking about it?"
- Share their journey with them. Weep when they weep. Laugh when they laugh.

- Touch is beneficial to most patients. It shows you still care.
- Try to be alone with the patient. Help patient verbalize fears. Enumerate various possibilities. Think and talk through them together clearly and rationally. "Pain control" their emotions.
- Help patient prepare mentally for the worst possible outcome. This discussion will give them calm and peace, renewed courage and determination to meet whatever the future holds, because they will have already verbally and mentally worked through it.
- Caution the patient about bargaining with God or making any rash promises.
- Include the patient in the decision making, health or family issues.
- Let patient preach their own sermon...regarding this crisis, their faith, their confidence and courage. This is about coping with their condition not succumbing to it.
- Help family accept that the patient may desire to change "cure" goals to "comfort" goals and to die in the most conducive setting for them.
- Bring their favorite meals in disposable containers, if they have no restrictions. Let them know what time to expect you and be there.
- Take their children out to give them all a break from this highly stressful situation.
- Help them with cleaning, dishes, laundry or grocery shopping.
- Decorate their room if it is near a holiday. Bring small gifts and flowers.
- Be creative. Bring books, encouraging words, cards, flowers, taped music, momentums of significant life ex-

periences, posters for the wall, snack baskets for patient's family.

- Send cards when you can't come and let them know they are still in your heart.
- Pray, pray, pray. Share uplifting scriptures.

MINISTERING TO THE DYING AND BEREAVED
(See chapter Support of Dying Patient, Death and Grief)

- Address your own fear of death before you attempt to minister effectively to dying patients and their families.
- Check with the nurse before seeing the patient.
- Ask for time alone with the patient. This may mean that you will have to ask their family to step out for a moment. This time to share with a "representative of God" may be critically needed by the dying patient.
- The fewer the words the better. "I'm sorry" is always appropriate. Be a "listening presence."
- Simple things like swabbing the patient's lips with a wet sponge stick, pulling up the sheet to keep the breeze off them, cool cloth on forehead, massage hands, feet, legs gently if appropriate or desired, can make a difference in their comfort level.
- Ask staff if it would be a convenient time for you to hold a service with the family.
- Remind family about the necessity of providing Durable Power of Health Care and Advance Directives, or state patient's wishes as they know them.
- Encourage the patient to have a Will or Trust drawn up while they are still able.
- Accept that all feelings of patient/family members as okay, even if irrational or "bad".

- Remind family that hearing is the last to go and that we want to keep positive and uplifting conversation around patient's bedside.
- Remind family that the patient has the right to express their feelings and emotions about their approaching death in their own way. And they have the right to be told the truth. They also have the right to die alone or with support.
- Protect the patient's dignity.
- Gather the family around the bed. Respect personal limits and boundaries.
- Remember....kids grieve. Seek them out. Include them. Patient has the right to have children around them if they so choose.
- Invite them to take time to talk alone to patient, especially if they need to ask for forgiveness or offer forgiveness.
- Ask them if they would like to sing some of the patient's favorite songs, or read some scriptures, (Ex. Psalm 23, Revelation 21:1-5). Share uplifting memories for the patient to hear. Take turns praying, or just you pray offering a word of thanksgiving for the life of the patient. You can encourage them to hold hands and say the Lord's Prayer together as you close.
- Remind family that grief comes in waves.
- Let them know that there may come a time when they will have to release the patient; give the patient permission to let go and stop fighting. Tell them to reassure the patient that they will be okay and that they will take care of each other. The patient has the right to not die alone or to die alone as they desire.

- Encourage the family to take care of themselves and keep their energy up. Take turns by the bedside, eat regular meals—even small amounts, get some rest—even short naps.
- Remind family and friends to be gentle with themselves and each other. Give each other grace; their emotions and reactions will be all over the map and they may not realize when they are acting "weird" or unreasonable. Be extra forgiving and overlooking.
- Be sure family has appropriate support, personally and with their families at home.
- If you are present at the time of death ensure that the sanctity of patient's body is respected.
- Let family know of your availability as you depart.

Support of Patient and Family during Dying, Death, and Grief

A young pastor came to my office badly shaken, crying, "Please help me. I've never had to deal with anything like this before." The pastor had been called to the Emergency Room after a car accident had taken the life of one of his parishioners, a young wife and mother. Two small children, an infant and toddler, would soon find out that Mommy wouldn't be coming home. The husband, not yet informed, was on his way to meet the pastor and then to view the body of his wife.

Among other things, I shared with this pastor that while it was okay to cry, a calm spiritual presence was one of the most effective ways of ministering to the suddenly bereaved. Just being present would fill an immense need for the husband. I alerted him that the husband might have many exclamatory remarks and may lose his composure. He may just need the pastor to hold him. A consoling method is often to keep repeating, "I'm sorry. I'm so sorry."

I also encouraged him not to make excuses for God or defend God. Questions and anger towards God would most likely be forthcoming. I suggested he reassure his parishioner that God's shoulders are big enough for any questions and that He can handle our anger.

For a pastor, the support of a dying patient can be one of the most difficult ministry arenas. For one thing, our culture denies death so rigorously. For another thing, pastors like to help solve problems and to have answers. A pastor may feel helpless when he comes face to face with death. Death involves helping with the acceptance of the fact and how to cope, not in solving the problem. Death involves walking with a grieving person, and crying with them. And a third reason it is difficult to be present during death and grieving is because it encompasses such an emotionally charged atmosphere.

You too may have deep insecurities about being present during the dying process and feel inadequate when called to the hospital into such an emotionally charged atmosphere. We all have had moments when we feel inadequate, ill prepared or over-zealous to minister and do not come through in the best way. Being prepared and equipped lowers the odds of failure.

Story: I was a fairly new chaplain responding to an emergency call. Hurrying into the Intensive Care Unit, I was instructed that a young woman was dying. I was needed to support her husband and brother. They were requesting a chaplain to come pray with them. In my haste to "do my job" I came to the bedside, announced who I was and said, "You requested prayer?" "Yes." After a few more words I began to pray. It never entered my mind to ask what their faith tradition was. I just prayed my little heart out to Jesus. After I said, "Amen," they began to chant. I was appalled, perplexed, and embarrassed. After that experience, I remembered to pray for guidance before responding to a need or ministering to those in distress.

Every person, every family, and every need is different. Go prepared by being prayed up and focused on your mission.

VISITING A DYING PERSON IN THE HOSPITAL

If you image yourself to be seriously ill or told that you are terminally ill, that you only had so long to live, what would you want someone to say to you? What would you want to talk about? What service(s)/ceremonies might you want to have at your bedside? It helps to take a moment and put yourself in someone else's shoes. When you have a sense of their feelings or needs your ministry and support will be more meaningful and effective.

Dying and grieving is a process. The process includes **denial, anger, bargaining,** and lastly **acceptance.** Sometimes people will fluctuate between these stages. When they come to acceptance, it opens them up to coping with their situation and usually perpetuates them getting their "business in order" or moving forward.

Having faith and praying for people to get well is something else entirely. As we trust in Him, we can be thankful that no one can interrupt God's perfect plan for the patient. His word promises that He will be our guide even unto death. (Psalms 48:14) When praying, do not project as a "faith healer". Ultimately we must accept that God has a plan and purpose for each life. While death is an interruption of God's perfect plan, that we were to live forever, it is a reality of the consequences of sin and our life on this earth. In Isaiah 57:1-2 we are instructed, "The righteous perish and no one ponders it in his heart; devout men are taken away, and no one understands that the righteous are taken away to be spared from evil. Those who walk uprightly enter into peace; and they find rest as they lie in death."

We do not know when it is the end of one's time on this earth. We can pray our heart, claim God's promises, and ask for God's will, that His destiny for the patient be fulfilled. In some cases it is okay if the patient chooses death. Be sensitive to the situation and to God's voice.

Here are some suggestions on how to communicate with the dying, and after death with the survivors.

PREPARATION FOR THE VISIT

- Pray for guidance before entering the room.
- Take with you scripture or inspirational material that is comforting, not preachy.
- Expect to see physical changes that can be shocking.
- Seek briefing from the family or from the hospital chaplain re: patient's condition.
- Stop at the Nursing Station first to ask if there's anything you should know.

MINISTERING TO ADULTS WHO ARE DYING

Your goal is to help the patient face death with dignity, confidence, calmness and peace.

- Knock first before entering.
- Ask if the patient would like a visit from you just then.
- Pray at his/her bedside out loud if the patient is comatose. (Touch and hearing are the last senses to go as we die.)
- Establish rapport. If the patient is alert, look into his/her eyes. Get close to the bed. Gently put your hand on the person's arm and explain your visit: "I'm here, (name), to pray with you." Sometimes small talk can ease tension,

but don't spend too much time there. Some mention of your congregation and how they are praying for the patient can be comforting.

- Encourage story telling. The patient needs to know that their life mattered; that they are leaving a legacy. This will help them find meaning and also help them "let go" of life.

- Ask the patient if there's anything they want from you and listen to the answer. You may hear, often between the lines, that they are fearful, angry at God, resigned, or guilty at leaving loved ones behind. There may even be denial. You don't have to fix or solve these feelings, just listen to them.

- Offer to help, if you feel qualified and comfortable, or find someone who would be able to help if practical concerns come up. (Such as the hospital's Social Worker). If the patient has any complaints of pain or discomfort, offer to call the nurse. Don't do anything yourself; even easy things such as raising or lowering their bed.

- Offer to pray. Offer scriptural readings. Offer whatever you feel would give comfort. (Sometimes even the gift of a cuddly stuffed toy is most gratefully accepted).

- Test the waters about their concept and acceptance of death by asking the question: "Where do you imagine you're going (name)?" If a person has been longing to talk but has held back because he has been fearful or because he doesn't want to upset loved ones, this can be a break in dammed up emotions. Listen. All emotions are okay. If a patient wants to know what's after death, you might be prepared to relate this information.

- Come prepared to offer sacraments to the patient if they are able/allowed to partake; if they want to have communion. Check first with the nurse. You don't want to start something sacred just to have it interrupted by medical procedures or visits.

- Bedside ceremonies can include scripture reading, song(s), memory sharing, prayer, and repeating the Lord's Prayer together, holding hands.
- Be sensitive to the patient's need to rest and sleep, not overstaying. It's often best to keep visits brief, but more frequent, than to spend an hour or longer visiting.
- Encourage forgiveness—of self, of others, even of God.
- Let the patient know that even when they feel alone, they are not. Remind them that their loved ones, the congregation, and you are praying for them and that God is always as close as their hearts.

See also chapter on Ministering to Different Populations, section Ministering to Critically Ill

MINISTERING TO CHILDREN WHO ARE DYING

- Check with parents to ascertain what the child has been told, and how the child has accepted the information. Honesty is best in most cases because children often feel they're not being told the truth. If parents have no objection, then ask some leading questions, such as "What do you think heaven is like,____?" This questioning can elicit a response that opens up a whole conversation that might reveal fear or confusion.
- Being the child's friend can be healing and comforting. Bring a stuffed animal if allowed, a big card that has been signed by all the kids from church; a child-type joke,

puzzles or a game to play. It's good to remember: until the moment of death, the patient is alive. Treat them so.

- Straight talk can be helpful when a dying child is concerned about their parents' ability to cope. For example, "Your parents love you so much. They know that you'll be okay, but they'll really, really miss you."
- Touch is important, so when appropriate a hand in theirs is comforting.
- Offer to read them a story that touches on death.
- Praying for children can be couched in terms of "talking with God." Start the conversation: "Dear Father God, I'm here with _____. As you know, he/she is very sick." This can help a young patient feel that God is a friend and will listen.

See Chapter 1, Visitation Etiquette; Preparation for the Visit—Age and Developmental Stages

MINISTERING TO THE FAMILY

- Remaining calm and being there for the family is what is most needed. Once the prognosis of death is obvious, loved ones often go through emotional turmoil, needing your presence and help as much as the dying patient. Anticipatory grief is common as they try to imagine what life will be like after the death.
- Listen. Not endeavoring to fix things, or to mitigate their grief. Speak with them outside of the patient's room, in a place that is "safe" in case they break down and need to cry. Encourage family members to cry together. No one needs to be strong. "Strong" isn't necessarily spiritual or reflective of their relationship with God.

- Assist where reconciliation is needed by being the bridge between the dying and their loved ones. While getting in the middle of a dispute isn't usually wise, you can sense when a little explanation of the other's behavior may help soften a seemingly intractable or highly charged situation.
- Encourage forgiveness promptly and whole-heartedly.
- Encourage expression of feelings and emotions. This is not the time to stuff them.

     Some are overwhelmed with the thought of loss. They feel abandoned by God. They wonder why when they have been so faithful and given so much of themselves for the church or ministry that God would allow this to happen. They question God and themselves. (**Isaiah 57:1-2** might be advantageous to share at this time.)

- Help them start planning for the funeral or memorial service.

WHAT TO AVOID

- Avoid joking or rushing on to a safer topic and not allowing people to be fully in their feelings. These are some of the ways people stay on the surface
- Avoid disregarding your own feelings. If you need to cry, feel sad, or grieve, do it.
- Avoid taking charge or "rescuing". No doubt the patient and the family need counseling, practical help with such things as funeral arrangements, and encouragement; but there is no short cut in dying or in grieving.
- Avoid platitudes. When in doubt, be silent and pray for guidance.

THE BEREAVED

Be sensitive and tolerant of the physical and emotional limits of the survivors, especially in the days immediately following the death. Feelings of loss and sadness, as well as the days of turmoil preceding death, cause fatigue. Encourage the family to respect what their body and mind are telling them. Nutrition is extremely important. Encourage daily balanced meals and regular rest; even naps if necessary.

DEATH OF ADULT PATIENTS
RESPONSE TO SUDDEN DEATH

- Pray first before you get there and get centered. You will be the lifeline to the shocked and grieving loved ones. Check in with the hospital chaplain or the nurses to get quick briefing.

- Connect with the survivors. A clasp of the hand or hug and the sentiment "I'm so very sorry," lets them know you're with them. Introduce yourself to family and friends unknown to you. When people are in shock, they may forget who you are, even if they've met you before. The fewer words the better. "I'm sorry" is always appropriate.

- Before family goes in to see body, check to see if the deceased is presentable (eyes closed, covered, wounds washed).

- Ask the loved ones if they want to see the patient ("Do you want to see your father now?"). Prepare them for any problems with the body, such as bruises, wounds and then ask them if they'd like your company. Your presence can be tremendously helpful. If they say "no", wait outside the door and let them know you will be there if they need you.

- Encourage the survivors to say goodbye if they are consumed with not having had the opportunity. Gently let them know that they can say goodbye now. Let them touch, kiss, or hold their deceased loved one.

- Bring comfort to the survivors by leading them in a brief heartfelt prayer. If appropriate hold their hands, grounding them with your touch. Ask if they would like to join you in the 'Lord's Prayer' at the conclusion of your personal prayer. While a shocked person might not be able to pray themselves, they are often grateful and comforted by you interceding for them. They might also gain comfort by repeating, with you, a prayer they are familiar with.

- Don't leave the survivor(s) alone at the hospital until you know what the plan is once they leave there. Who plans to be with them at home? Who will pick them up and drive them back home?

- Excuse yourself and reassure family of your continual prayers and thoughts in their behalf. If you stay around when the family just wants to be alone together and would rather you aren't present, grieving becomes more difficult and aggravates an already sensitive situation where feelings of anger may be present.

- Alert your congregation if you have received permission. Hopefully you'll already have services/resources in place to help the survivors cope.

- Keep in touch. If the survivors aren't of your congregation, you might refer them to helpful services or support groups. Make a follow-up call to let them know you care.

RESPONSE TO EXPECTED DEATH

- Because a survivor may have undergone a lot of anticipatory grief already, the actual death may be somewhat of a relief; especially if the patient was suffering a lot. They could still be in a state of shock, though.
- Offer to pray, holding hands if appropriate.
- Stay with them.
- Ask them how you can be the most help to them.
- Don't leave them alone. Make sure someone will pick them up and be with them at home.

PRENATAL DEATH *(See Chapter Healing and Deliverance Scriptures—Heading-Infant Death)*

- Grieving is difficult because no memories are built up and friends and family expect them to get right over it.
- Parents, especially the mother, may suffer from "empty arms syndrome." Some mothers are thankful for a teddy bear to hold and cry into; others are angered by the thought that a stuffed bear could take the place of their lost child.
- Actively assist parents through this time:
  - by suggesting a naming ceremony. If possible provide the spiritual meaning of baby's name and the text. Write it in a card so they can take it with them. (See "The Name Book" by Dorothy Astoria ISBN 1-55661-982-0)
  - by having them diaper and dress the baby.
  - by making hand and foot prints on craft paper or clay molds for family members. (Nursing staff usually has all of this available and will assist you.)

Story: Several years ago, I had an experience while ministering to the grieving that will be forever etched in my mind. Families had been gathering at a special function. Excited children were running around, enjoying each others' company, fully engrossed in their play. Two families arrived together. They were in a large truck with a number of items to unload. In the short moment that the driver stopped to receive instructions, one of the young boys jumped on the back of the truck. When the truck started moving, it lurched, throwing the child onto the road. Before anyone even knew he was there, the driver, backing up, ran over the small boy.

This precious little guy was immediately taken to the hospital, but was found dead on arrival. As the hospital chaplain, I was called to the Emergency Room to meet the family as they arrived. When the child's mother heard the news, she fell on the floor wailing, writhing in pain, clutching the floor, and screaming. None of us knew what to do.

My heart was breaking as I witnessed her anguish. I laid down on the floor, on my back, next to her, and took her in my arms and held her. She sobbed and sobbed, hanging on to me for dear life.

When she was ready, we transitioned her to where her son was. She held and rocked him for almost four hours. I finally asked a friend to go to this mother's home and bring back her son's favorite blanket and toy. When she returned with them, I helped the mother wrap her son in the blanket and told her that it was almost time for her to leave him with me.

I would like to suggest that pastors, or spiritual care representatives, must be willing to do whatever it takes to minister to such broken-hearted ones. Share the journey with those experiencing loss. Words are not as necessary as your presence and your love.

DEATH OF CHILDREN

There often is a devastating feeling of guilt—that the parent wasn't able to protect his child or save him. Thus, added to grief are strong emotions of not being adequate. If these emotions disrupt a survivor's life for more than three to six months then professional counseling, both psychological and spiritual, is recommended.

- The death of a child often triggers deep emotions in hospital staff and maybe in you. Don't be ashamed of tears.

- You might have to advocate for parents with the staff, for a little more time before parting with their loved one.

- At the hospital, encourage parents to say goodbye in whatever way they want. Holding the child, getting a clipping of hair--these can be particularly comforting in the moment and in the future as well.

- Calling them several weeks after their child's death to either offer them your services or make a referral is a next step.

WHAT NOT TO SAY:

- **At least you have other children.**
- **You are young, you can have other children.**
- **God doesn't make mistakes. He has a reason.**
- **God wants your baby more than you do.**
- **It was God's will.**

Grief

Story: Through my life I have suffered a number of losses. My little sister died when she was seven. I was eleven. She died of measles that developed into pneumonia then encephalitis. The following year my father died of a heart attack. Then I lost my grandmother from cancer, had a couple of miscarriages, lost my first granddaughter from SIDS (Sudden Infant Death), my 25-year-old son died in an automobile accident, lost my husband from divorce, my step-father from congestive heart failure and chronic obstructive pulmonary disease, and three women friends that were like sisters to me; all of Cancer. My most recent loss was my father-in-law from a heart attack.

In each case I reacted differently. When my sister died I tried to be strong for my mother. I didn't allow myself to grieve. When my father died my parents were in the middle of a divorce. I was able to grieve for him and for my little sister. His death had been unexpected. For years, I carried around guilt for how I had reacted to him the day before his death. When I lost my son I took care of my family, but very mechanically. I couldn't remember how I had gone from the living room to the kitchen. When my granddaughter died I was in a fog but present to grieve with and support our children. After raising seven sons, losing the first little girl in our family seemed unimaginable.

When grieving, one might feel sad one minute and then find themselves laughing at a memory. They might want people around them and the next minute want to be alone. They may go from angry to loving and from capable to incapable.

The most powerful thing for people to do is embrace their grief. It will come in waves and they just have to ride them out. Encourage them to be gentle with themselves and with those grieving with them. In many cases, they will be unaware of how they are presenting.

HELP THOSE WORKING THROUGH GRIEF:
- acknowledge/accept the reality of the loss.
- express the emotions of grief; these are anger, denial, acceptance.
- acknowledge feelings of ambivalence. Caregivers for chronically or terminally ill patients that have struggled with anticipatory grief may face feelings of guilt and will need to work through it. (This could be guilt of "thankfulness that this is finally over", or how they treated or abandoned patient, or how they began looking towards a new life/future before patient died.)
- help resolve feelings of ambivalence. (This takes place as family parts with personal items of the deceased member. Often difficult because they do not want to let go and move on: exhibited most by family members overwrought with guilt. People fight change, even if it is positive change.)
- let go and move on. Look towards the future.

As a pastor or spiritual leader, it is vital that you give the family permission to move toward their grief and heal. Reconciling grief does not happen quickly. Remember that the death of someone loved changes the lives of the survivors forever. Some feel guilty about moving on. It helps to be granted permission.

GRIEVING CHILDREN

- Ministering to children whose family member has died requires considerable sensitivity. The children need to be included. If they don't ask, bring up the subject. They may think it is not okay to talk about it. They will have many questions which will come up again and again.

- If the child is at the hospital, describe to them what the patient looks like and that they don't look like themselves. Explain that the patient has a tube in their mouth and tubes going to their arm. Prepare the child. If they are going to the funeral home, explain. Do not ask the child if they want to see. The child will wonder what they shouldn't see or why they shouldn't go.

- Let them know that it is okay to be sad and cry. Allow them to grieve. It helps bring closure to the separation. Explain that death is a natural part of the life cycle.

- Some children may laugh. This is not abnormal. They simply don't understand; they are uncomfortable and don't know what to do. Sometimes they are afraid to cry for fear they will not stop. Give them time. Do not make them feel guilty nor accuse them of having no feelings. Be patient.

- Reassure child that they are not responsible. Nothing they thought, said, or how they acted caused this.
- Let them know that they will see adults crying too.
- **Don't** tell them Jesus needed more angels in heaven.
- **Don't** say (s)he just went to sleep and didn't wake up. (The child will be afraid to go to sleep.)
- **Don't** make heaven sound so delightful that they want to go out and get hit by a car too, so they can be where mom or dad is.
- **Do use** natural life cycles from nature, such as fallen leaves, to explain the process of life and death. Some have also used balloons and let them float away to explain that death is a lot like the balloon. You can't go where it is going now, but you can remember it when you were playing with it.
- With young children, it is comforting to "remember when" and share memories with them.

GRIEVING TEENS

- Teens deal with grief with their peers. They support each other.
- They distract through technology.
- Make sure they are included, consulted, and have an opportunity to share.
- Reassure them that it is alright to cry. Invite them to let out their tears; that if they keep them bottled up inside it can make them sick.
- **Let them know that they don't have to be strong for anyone. That everyone needs to express their heartache, and it is best for everyone to cry together.**

MEANINGFUL FUNERALS/MEMORIAL SERVICES

- Meaningful services include all close family members in the planning process.

- It is important to remember that the services are for the survivors acknowledging the death of someone they love. It's a way for them to focus on those things that were noteworthy about their loved one. It opens the opportunity for support from caring people.

- Each service can be unique and distinctive according to the needs of the particular family. Comfort and meaning from traditional ceremonies can still reflect the unique personality of the family and the person who died. Adding personal touches to even traditional services can make the service one that will be remembered and appreciated. (See following examples.)

- Give the family the freedom to ask friends and other family members to be involved in the service. They can share responsibilities or participate in activities such as special reading, writing and reading the eulogy, special music, or inviting attendees to share memories.

- Encourage the family and close friends to view the body before entering the service. Many people find this helps them acknowledge the reality of the death. It also provides a way to say goodbye. There is nothing morbid or wrong about this practice.

- Another effective and consoling goodbye gift is to have a bouquet of roses or other preferred flowers at the graveside. Pass them out to family members to lie on top of the casket. You can invite them to place flowers there at the end of your service. You can also invite them to pray a favorite prayer or cherish a memory as they place their flower.

- Encourage survivors to embrace their feelings and openly express them. There is no shame in crying.
- The service should also reflect the spirituality of the families and the deceased. If there is any question what direction to take, lean towards the spirituality of the deceased. (Unless they were not Christian and you have an audience of many Christians or seekers.) Help survivors to find comfort in their faith through the service.
- Frequently when a loved one dies, the survivors might find themselves questioning their faith, and the very meaning of life and death. This is natural. Encourage the search for meaning. Do not let others dismiss this journey with clichéd responses, such as," It was God's will." Or "Think of what you still have to be thankful for."
- Make use of memories during the service. Fun, personal memories can be included in the eulogy to make it more interesting, and draw more people in. Memories are part of the best legacies that exist after the death of someone loved. Stress the word "legacy" and what the deceased is leaving behind for the family to hang on to and live out in their lives. Ask those attending the funeral to share their most special memory of the person who died.
- Some people are reticent about sharing in a group setting. Encourage sharing at the reception following. Encourage visitors to share particular memories of the deceased that would become a treasure to the hearer.
- If you are not familiar with the deceased, after reading or hearing the eulogy and listening to the stories shared, a nice thing to say is," I wish I had known _____. I think we would have been good friends.

g by reading the poem "The Dash"
ttp://www.notalone.co.nz/the-dash-
make an appeal.

y small box (like jewelry box-brace-
in shiny gold paper. Tell them, "It
is a 'Memory Box' not to be opened but to remind
them of cherished memories".

• Suggest they plant a tree or flowering shrub in their
yard in memory of their loved one, or establish a
Memory Garden area.

• For some, it is beneficial to have them write the deceased a letter. Encourage them to share their feelings, even to say, "I'm angry with you for leaving
me." Have them write memories, words of thanks,
dreams that will go unfulfilled, and their love. They
can place this letter in the casket, put it away until
the first year anniversary of death, or until they want
to reread it, if ever.

CAUTION: Do not assume that people will want to memorialize
the date of death. Some families would rather not be reminded of
this heart ache every year. They will never forget their loved one.
There will be memories forever tucked in their minds and heart.
They will see their loved one in the faces and mannerisms of other
family members. But to have an appointed day for grieving is
debilitating to them.

Self Care

TAKING CARE OF YOURSELF

Do you take time for yourself to be refreshed and renewed, revived and regenerated? Do you take time to refill your cup, so you can continue to give? Do you honor yourself and your Creator by self care? "Don't you know that you yourselves are God's temple and that God's Spirit lives in you?" (I Corinthians 3:16)

This chapter is a gentle reminder to take care of yourself, so that you don't burn out and then find yourself dropping out of the serving roles you fill. Ministering to your hospitalized parishioners is a needed and relevant service. Many patients feel/believe that they don't matter to the pastor if he/she doesn't personally come by to check on them. They might think of themselves as a "case" a "problem" a "project". If they don't make it on your visitation list, they weren't your priority.

An alternative to you visiting is to establish and train a Hospital Visitation Team. This would be good self care, but the truth is, it might precipitate a drop in your membership/attendance. After all, in the patient's eyes, no one can take your place. Here are some better suggestions for taking care of you!

DEBRIEFING AFTER A VISIT

- Get alone and pray to God for guidance, for clarity, for relief of a burden. Leave the responsibility for the patient's healing in His hands. Give yourself to God too.
- Talk to someone; maybe the hospital chaplain, about a visit or situation that upsets you. In other words, don't just swallow it. The chaplain will advocate for fair treatment, help bring about resolve regarding your concerns, or put you in contact with people that can help you. Debrief, and do it soon.
- Assess yourself. How did you minister to patient? Did you go in your own strength or empowered by God as His instrument?
- Check any negative self talk. Change it to positive self talk. For example, if you find that you are berating yourself for not having said or done something better, immediately say to yourself something like, "I did the best I could at that time. I'm learning and getting better each time I make a visit".
- Forgive yourself for making any mistakes.

SPIRITUAL AND EMOTIONAL SELF CARE

- Pray, meditate and praise systematically. God "inhabits the praises of His people." Praise dispels the enemy. Trust in God.
- Express gratitude. It's amazing how good this feels.
- Study Scripture and other inspiring works regularly.
- Take alone time for honest self-reflection, being aware of your issues, feelings, or needs. A spiritual seclusion would be wonderful; quiet time--quiet place.

- Spend some time in nature.
- Journal. This is a good way to ease stress. It's a method of illuminating introspection.
- Reward yourself often with something you like to do or by being with people you enjoy. It is okay to put yourself first sometimes.
- Change your routine.
- Develop interests outside of your ministry.
- Laugh, play, practice feeling joyful, focus on happy things.
- Don't compromise your own convictions, insights, or opinions.
- Allow yourself to be loved and taken care of. You don't have to do all the giving.
- Request support. Talk, identify, express and release your feelings. It's okay to cry.
- Beware of compassion fatigue.
- Spend time with family and friends, but feel free to say "no" if you feel like being alone.
- Maintain healthy boundaries.

PHYSICAL SELF CARE

- Exercise regularly and get plenty of sunshine. You've probably heard all this before, but experiment with what will work for you. Walk, jog, bike, swim regularly every week. You will notice that you will feel better physically and be uplifted emotionally.
- Get sufficient rest. Participate in relaxation exercises to reduce stress.
- Eat healthy. Understand your nutritional needs. Read a book about proper nutrition and preventative health. Eat more whole foods, less junk foods and see how you

begin to feel. Treat your body like the temple it is. Increased energy could be the payoff.

- Drink plenty of pure water.
- Practice temperance.

To catch a cold occasionally is something most of us face. If you're getting sick a lot though, it might be your body/mind telling you that it needs some downtime. Take some time off. Definitely **don't** go to the hospital if you're not feeling well. If necessary, get a physical exam to rule out any complications.

ARE YOUR NEEDS BEING MET?

- You aren't going to last in the service role if you're frustrated or unhappy. For instance, if you feel you're being overworked and undervalued by someone in authority over you, or by your church family, you're certainly not in a win-win situation. This can lead to resentment and burnout.
- Be clear. What are your needs? What do you want? How can you get it? Who can help?
- Talk with a counselor, chaplain, another pastor, friend, or loved one about your feelings. They could help you identify how to change. Allow yourself the freedom to disregard their advice and follow your own, change your mind or choose a different course of action; but do something to care for you.
- Are you receiving, as well as giving? Practice self care so you have something to give others.

WARNING SIGNS OF COMPASSION FATIGUE

Symptoms vary, but the following red flags may indicate that you have compassion fatigue. The following warning signs were taken from the article *Overcoming Compassion Fatigue* by John-Henry Pfifferling, PhD, and Kay Gilley, MS.

- Anger
- Blaming
- Chronic lateness
- Hopelessness
- High self-expectations
- Low self-esteem
- Apologize for being yourself
- Increased irritability
- Feel guilty about what you desire
- Less ability to feel joy
- Addictive, abusive, or victim behaviors
- Appetite or sleep disturbances, nightmares
- Diminished sense of personal accomplishment
- Depression, despair, sadness, uncontrollable tears
- Inability to maintain balance of empathy and objectivity
- Exhaustion (physical or emotional) You've drained your strength for others.
- Stress-related illnesses, frequent headaches, gastrointestinal complaints, hypertension, etc

Hospital Ministry— Healing & Deliverance Scriptures

The Bible is an inspiring, encouraging, and reassuring resource when dealing with sickness and suffering. There is power in the word of God. Albeit we don't understand, God has a purpose in allowing sickness and suffering. He cares for our needs and carries our burdens. Pain and suffering can lead us closer to God. He answers our "Prayer of Faith" according to His divine will. He will give sufficient grace for every trial.

The following scriptures have been quoted from the New King James Version unless otherwise noted.

Abandonment

Isa 49:15-16 Can a woman forget her nursing child, and not have compassion on the son of her womb? Surely they may forget, yet I will not forget you. 16 See, I have inscribed you on the palms of My hands; your walls are continually before Me.

Abuse

<u>Zeph 3:15, 19-20</u> The LORD has taken away the judgments against you, He has cast out your enemies. The King of Israel, the LORD, is in your midst; you shall fear evil no more. 19 Behold, at that time I will deal with all your oppressors. I will save the lame and gather the outcast, and I will change their shame into praise and renown in all the earth. 20 At that time I will bring you home, at the time when I gather you together; yea, I will make you renowned and praised among all the peoples of the earth, when I restore your fortunes before your eyes," says the LORD. (RSV)

Afflictions

<u>Ex 3:7-8</u> And Jehovah said, I have surely seen the affliction of My people…and have heard their cry…for I know their sorrows; 8 So I have come down to deliver them. (ASV)

<u>Isa 53:4-5</u> Surely He has borne our griefs and carried our sorrows; yet we esteemed Him stricken, smitten by God, and afflicted. 5 But He was wounded for our transgressions, He was bruised for our iniquities; The chastisement for our peace was upon Him, and by His stripes we are **healed**.

<u>Mt 4:24</u> Then His fame went throughout all Syria; and they brought to Him all sick people who were afflicted with various diseases and torments, and those who were demon-possessed, epileptics, and paralytics; and He **healed** them.

<u>Mk 3:10</u> For He **healed** many, so that as many as had afflictions pressed about Him to touch Him.

Mk 5:34 And He said to her, "Daughter, your faith has made you well. Go in peace, and be **healed** of your affliction."
Acts 7:10 and rescued him out of all his afflictions, (RSV)

Acts 9:34 And Peter said to him, "Aeneas, Jesus the Christ **heals** you. Arise and make your bed." Then he arose immediately.

Alcohol/Addictions
Pr 20:1 Wine is a mocker, strong drink a brawler; and whoever is led astray by it is not wise.

Pr 23:29-35 Who has woe? Who has sorrow? Who has strife? Who has complaining? Who has wounds without cause? Who has redness of eyes? 30 Those who tarry long over wine, those who go to try mixed wine. 31 Do not look at wine when it is red, when it sparkles in the cup and goes down smoothly. 32 At the last it bites like a serpent, and stings like an adder. 33 Your eyes will see strange things, and your mind utter perverse things. 34 You will be like one who lies down in the midst of the sea, like one who lies on the top of a mast. 35 "They struck me," you will say, "but I was not hurt; they beat me, but I did not feel it. When shall I awake? I will seek another drink." (RSV)

Isa 24:9 They shall not drink wine with a song. Strong drink is bitter to those who drink it.

Ankles

<u>Acts 3:7-8</u> And He took him by the right hand and lifted him up, and immediately his feet and ankle bones received strength. 8 So he, leaping up, stood and walked and entered the temple with them--walking, leaping, and praising God.

Backsliding

<u>Hos 14:4</u> I will **heal** their backsliding, I will love them freely, for My anger has turned away from him.

Barren

<u>Gen 15:2-4</u> But Abram said, "Lord GOD, what will You give me, seeing I go childless,..." 3 Then Abram said, "Look, You have given me no offspring; indeed one born in my house is my heir!" 4 And behold, the word of the LORD came to him, saying, "This one shall not be your heir, but one who will come from your own body shall be your heir."

<u>Gen 20:17</u> So Abraham prayed to God, and God **healed** Abimelech, his wife, and his female servants. Then they bore children;

<u>Ex 23:25-26</u> So you shall serve the LORD your God, and He will bless your bread and your water. And I will take sickness away from the midst of you. 26 No one shall suffer miscarriage or be barren in your land; I will fulfill the number of your days.

Blind

Isa 29:18 In that day the deaf shall hear the words of a book, and out of their gloom and darkness the eyes of the blind shall see. (RSV)

Mt 12:22 Then one was brought to Him who was demon-possessed, blind and mute; and He **healed** him, so that the blind and mute man both spoke and saw.

Mt 13:16 But blessed are your eyes for they see, and your ears for they hear; (spiritual eyes)

Mt 15:30 Then great multitudes came to Him, having with them the lame, blind, mute, maimed, and many others; and they laid them down at Jesus' feet, and He **healed** them.

Mt 21:14 Then the blind and the lame came to Him in the temple, and He **healed** them.

Mk 8:22-25 Then He came to Bethsaida, and they brought a blind man to Him, and begged Him to touch him. 23 So He took the blind man by the hand and led him out of the town. And when He had spit on his eyes and put His hands on him, He asked him if he saw anything. 24 And he looked up and said, "I see men like trees, walking." 25 Then He put His hands on his eyes again and made him look up. And he was restored and saw everyone clearly.

Lk 4:18 The Spirit of the LORD *is* upon Me, because He has anointed Me to preach the gospel to the poor; He has sent Me to **heal** the brokenhearted, to proclaim liberty to the captives and recovery of sight to the blind, to set at liberty those who are oppressed;

Jn 9:7 saying to him, "Go, wash in the pool of Siloam" (which means Sent). So he went and washed and came back seeing. (RSV)

Blood Transfusion
Lev 17:11 For the life of the flesh is in the blood:

Boils
Isa 38:21 Now Isaiah had said, "Let them take a lump of figs, and apply it as a poultice on the boil, and he shall recover."

2 Ki 20:7 Then Isaiah said, "Take a lump of figs." So they took and laid it on the boil, and he recovered.

Bones
Ps 6:2 Have mercy on me, O LORD, for I *am* weak; O LORD, **heal** me, for my bones are troubled.

Pr 3:5-8 Trust in the LORD with all your heart, and lean not on your own understanding; 6 In all your ways acknowledge Him, and He shall direct your paths. 7 Do not be wise in your own eyes; Fear the LORD and depart from evil. 8 It will be health to your flesh, and strength to your bones.

Pr 16:24 Pleasant words *are like* a honeycomb, sweetness to the soul and **health** to the bones.

Brokenhearted

Ps 34:18 The LORD is near to the brokenhearted, and saves the crushed in spirit.

Ps 147:3 He **heals** the brokenhearted, and binds up their wounds.

Isa 61:1 The Spirit of the Lord GOD is upon me, because the LORD has anointed me to bring good tidings to the afflicted; He has sent me to bind up the brokenhearted, to proclaim liberty to the captives, and the opening of the prison to those who are bound.

Bruise

Isa 30:26 In that day the LORD binds up the bruise of His people and **heals** the stroke of their wound.

Crippled

Acts 4:9,14,22 If we are being called to account today for an act of kindness shown to a cripple and are asked how he was **healed,** 14 and seeing the man who had been **healed** standing with them, they could say nothing against it. 22 For the man was over forty years old on whom this miracle of **healing** had been performed.

Acts 14:8,9 ...there sat a man crippled in his feet, who was lame from birth and had never walked. 9 This man heard Paul speaking. Paul, observing him intently and seeing that he had faith to be **healed,**

Deaf

Isa 29:18 In that day the deaf shall hear the words of a book, and out of their gloom and darkness the eyes of the blind shall see. (RSV)

Mt 13:16 But blessed are your eyes for they see, and your ears for they hear; (spiritual ears)

Mk 7:37 And they were astonished beyond measure, saying, "He has done all things well. He makes both the deaf to hear and the mute to speak."

Death (of Children Facing)

Gen 21:16-21 Then she went and sat down across from him at a distance of about a bowshot; for she said to herself, "Let me not see the death of the boy." So she sat opposite him, and lifted her voice and wept. 17 And God heard the voice of the lad. Then the angel of God called to Hagar out of heaven, and said to her, "What ails you, Hagar? Fear not, for God has heard the voice of the lad where he is. 18 Arise, lift up the lad and hold him with your hand, for I will make him a great nation." 19 Then God opened her eyes, and she saw a well of water. And she went and filled the skin with water, and gave the lad a drink. 20 So God was with the lad; and he grew and dwelt in the wilderness, and became an archer. 21 He dwelt in the Wilderness of Paran; and his mother took a wife for him from the land of Egypt. *Use with:*

Mt 19:14 But Jesus said, "Let the little children come to Me, and do not forbid them; for of such is the kingdom of heaven."

I Kings 20-23

Death (see also Life)

2Sam 22:2-7 And he said: "The LORD is my rock and my fortress and my deliverer; 3 The God of my strength, in Whom I will trust; My shield and the horn of my salvation, my stronghold and my refuge; my Savior, You save me from violence. 4 I will call upon the LORD, who is worthy to be praised; so shall I be saved from my enemies. 5 When the waves of death surrounded me, the floods of ungodliness made me afraid. 6 The sorrows of Sheol surrounded me; the snares of death confronted me. 7 In my distress I called upon the LORD, and cried out to my God; He heard my voice from His temple, and my cry entered His ears."

2Ki 20:5,8 Return and tell Hezekiah the leader of My people, 'Thus says the LORD, the God of David your father: "I have heard your prayer, I have seen your tears; surely I will **heal** you." On the third day you shall go up to the house of the LORD. 8 And Hezekiah said to Isaiah, "What *is* the sign that the LORD will **heal** me, and that I shall go up to the house of the LORD the third day?"

Job 19:25-27 For I know that my Redeemer lives, and He shall stand at last on the earth; 26 And after my skin is destroyed, this I know, that in my flesh I shall see God, 27 Whom I shall see for myself, and my eyes shall behold, and not another. How my heart yearns within me!

Ps 30:2 O LORD my God, I cried out to You, and You **healed** me.

Ps 48:14 For this is God, Our God forever and ever; He will be our guide *even* to death.

Ps 49:15 But God will redeem my soul from the power of the grave, for He shall receive me.

Ps 68:19-20 Blessed be the Lord, Who daily loads us with benefits, the God of our salvation! *Selah* 20 Our God is the God of salvation; and to GOD the Lord belongs escape from death.

Ps 103:3-4 Who forgives all your iniquities, Who **heals** all your diseases, Who redeems your life from destruction, Who crowns you with loving kindness and tender mercies,

Ps 107:18-20 Their soul abhorred all manner of food, and they drew near to the gates of death. 19 Then they cried out to the LORD in their trouble, and He saved them out of their distresses. 20 He sent His word and **healed** them, and delivered (rescued) *them* from their destructions (the grave).

Ps 116:1-9 I love the LORD, because He has heard my voice and my supplications. 2 Because He has inclined His ear to me.

Therefore I will call upon Him as long as I live. 3 The pains of death surrounded me, and the pangs of Sheol laid hold of me; I found trouble and sorrow. 4 Then I called upon the name of the LORD: "O LORD, I implore You, deliver my soul!" 5 Gracious is the LORD, and righteous; Yes, our God is merciful. 6 The LORD preserves the simple; I was brought low, and He saved me. 7 Return to your rest, O my soul, for the LORD has dealt bountifully with you. 8 For You have delivered my soul from death, my eyes from tears, and my feet from falling. 9 I will walk before the LORD in the land of the living.

Ps 118:17-18 I shall not die, but live, and declare the works of the LORD. 18 The LORD has chastened me severely, but He has not given me over to death.

Ps 119:116-7, 154 Uphold me according to Your word, that I may live; and do not let me be ashamed of my hope. 117 Hold me up, and I shall be safe, and I shall observe Your statutes continually. 154 Plead my cause and redeem me; revive me according to Your word.

Pr 18:21 Death and life are in the power of the tongue, and those who love it will eat its fruit.

Isa 25:8-9 He will swallow up death forever, and the Lord GOD will wipe away tears from all faces; The rebuke of His people He will take away from all the earth; for the LORD has spoken. 9 And it will be said in that day: "Behold, this is our God; we have waited for Him, and He will save us. This is the LORD; we have waited for Him; we will be glad and rejoice in His salvation."

Isa 57:1-2 The righteous perishes, and no man takes it to heart; merciful (devout) men are taken away, while no one considers that the righteous is taken away from evil (calamity). 2 He shall enter into peace; they shall rest in their beds, each one walking in his uprightness.

Hos13:14 I will ransom them from the power of the grave; I will redeem them from death. O Death, I will be your plagues! O Grave, I will be your destruction! Pity is hidden from My eyes.

Mk 5:23 and begged Him earnestly, saying, "My little daughter lies at the point of death. Come and lay Your hands on her, that she may be **healed**, and she will live."

Lu 7:3,7,10 So when he heard about Jesus, he sent elders of the Jews to Him, pleading with Him to come and **heal** his servant. 7 "Therefore I did not even think myself worthy to come to You. But say the word, and my servant will be **healed**. 10 Then the men who had been sent returned to the house and found the servant well.

Joh 3:16 For God so loved the world that He gave His only begotten Son, that whosoever believes in Him should not perish but have everlasting life.

Jn 4:47 When he heard that Jesus had come out of Judea into Galilee, he went to Him and implored Him to come down and **heal** his son, for he was at the point of death.

Rom 8:38-39 For I am persuaded that neither death nor life, nor angels nor principalities nor powers, nor things present nor things to come, 39 nor height nor depth, nor any other created thing, shall be able to separate us from the love of God which is in Christ Jesus our Lord.

Heb 5:7-8 who, in the days of His flesh, when He had offered up prayers and supplications, with vehement cries and tears to Him who was able to save Him from death, and was heard because of His godly fear, 8 though He was a Son, yet He learned obedience by the things which He suffered.

I Pet 1:3 Blessed be the God and Father of our Lord Jesus Christ, who according to His abundant mercy has begotten us again to a living hope through the resurrection of Jesus Christ from the dead,

Rev 3:10 Because you have kept My command to persevere, I also will keep you from the hour of trial which shall come upon the whole world, to test those who dwell on the earth.

Rev 14:13 Then I heard a voice from heaven saying to me, "Write: 'Blessed are the dead who die in the Lord from now on.'" "Yes," says the Spirit, "that they may rest from their labors, and their works follow them."

Death—Supportive Readings at Time of
(See the following section on Ministering Helps)

Deliverance

Ps 3:8 Deliverance belongs to the LORD; thy blessing be upon thy people!

Isa 61:1 The Spirit of the Lord GOD *is* upon Me, because the LORD has anointed Me to preach good tidings to the poor; He has sent Me to **heal** the brokenhearted, to proclaim liberty to the captives, and the opening of the prison to *those who are* bound;

Mt 4:24 Then His fame went throughout all Syria; and they brought to Him all sick people who were afflicted with various diseases and torments, and those who were demon-possessed, epileptics, and paralytics; and He **healed** them.

Mt 8:16 When evening had come, they brought to Him many who were demon-possessed. And He cast out the spirits with a word, and **healed** all who were sick,

Mt 10:1 And when He had called His twelve disciples to *Him,* He gave them power *over* unclean spirits, to cast them out, and to **heal** all kinds of sickness and all kinds of disease.

Mt 10:8 **Heal** the sick, cleanse the lepers, raise the dead, cast out demons. Freely you have received, freely give.

Mt 12:22 Then one was brought to Him who was demon-possessed, blind and mute; and He **healed** him, so that the blind and mute man both spoke and saw.

Mt 15:28 Then Jesus answered and said to her, "O woman, great *is* your faith! Let it be to you as you desire." And her daughter was **healed** from that very hour.

Mk 1:34 Then He **healed** many who were sick with various diseases, and cast out many demons; and He did not allow the demons to speak, because they knew Him.

Mk 3:15 and to have power to **heal** sicknesses and to cast out demons:

Mk 5:8, 9, 12,13 For He said to him, "Come out of the man, unclean spirit!" 9 Then He asked him, "What is your name?" And he answered, saying, "My name is Legion; for we are many." 12 So all the demons begged Him, saying, "Send us to the swine, that we may enter them." 13 And at once Jesus gave them permission. Then the unclean spirits went out and entered the swine (there were about two thousand);

Mk 6:13 And they cast out many demons, and anointed with oil many who were sick, and **healed** *them.*

Mk 7:25-30 For a woman whose young daughter had an unclean spirit heard about Him, and she came and fell at His feet. 26 The woman was a Greek, a Syro-Phoenician by birth, and she kept asking Him to cast the demon out of her daughter. 27 But Jesus said to her, "Let the children be filled first, for it is not good to take the children's bread and throw it to the little dogs." 28 And she answered and said to Him, "Yes, Lord, yet even the little dogs under the table eat from the children's crumbs." 29 Then He said to her, "For this saying go your way; the demon has gone out of your daughter." 30 And when she had come to her house, she found the demon gone out, and her daughter lying on the bed.

Lk 4:18 The Spirit of the LORD *is* upon Me, because He has anointed Me to preach the gospel to *the* poor; He has sent Me to heal the brokenhearted, to proclaim liberty to *the* captives and recovery of sight to *the* blind, to set at liberty those who are oppressed;

Lk 6:18 as well as those who were tormented with unclean spirits. And they were **healed**.

Lk 8:2 and certain women who had been **healed** of evil spirits and infirmities--Mary called Magdalene, out of whom had come seven demons,

Lk 8:36 They also who had seen *it* told them by what means he who had been demon-possessed was **healed**.

Lk 9:42 And as he was still coming, the demon threw him down and convulsed *him*. Then Jesus rebuked the unclean spirit, **healed** the child, and gave him back to his father.

Acts 5:16 Also a multitude gathered from the surrounding cities to Jerusalem, bringing sick people and those who were tormented by unclean spirits, and they were all **healed**.

Acts 10:38 how God anointed Jesus of Nazareth with the Holy Spirit and with power, who went about doing good and **healing** all who were oppressed by the devil, for God was with Him.

Diseases

<u>Ex 15:26</u> and said, "If you diligently heed the voice of the LORD your God and do what is right in His sight, give ear to His commandments and keep all His statutes, I will put none of the diseases on you which I have brought on the Egyptians; for I *am* the LORD who **heals** you."

<u>Deut. 7:11,12,15</u> Therefore you shall keep the commandment, the statutes, and the judgments which I command you today, to observe them. 12 Then it shall come to pass, because you listen to these judgments, and keep and do them, that the LORD your God will keep with you the covenant and the mercy which He swore to your fathers. 15 And the LORD will take away from you all sickness, and will afflict you with none of the terrible diseases of Egypt which you have known, but will lay them on all those who hate you.

<u>Ps 103:3</u> Who forgives all your iniquities, Who **heals** all your diseases,

<u>Mt 4:23</u> And Jesus went about all Galilee, teaching in their synagogues, preaching the gospel of the kingdom, and **healing** all kinds of sickness and all kinds of disease among the people.

<u>Mt 8:16-17</u> When evening had come, they brought to Him many who were demon-possessed. And He cast out the spirits with a word, and **healed** all who were sick, 17 that it might be fulfilled which was spoken by Isaiah the prophet, saying: "He Himself took our infirmities and bore our sicknesses."

<u>Mt 9:35</u> Then Jesus went about all the cities and villages, teaching in their synagogues, preaching the gospel of the kingdom, and **healing** every sickness and every disease among the people.

<u>Mt 10:1</u> And when He had called His twelve disciples to Him, He gave them power *over* unclean spirits, to cast them out, and to **heal** all kinds of sickness and all kinds of disease.

<u>Mk 1:33-34</u> And the whole city was gathered together at the door. 34 Then He **healed** many who were sick with various diseases, and cast out many demons; and He did not allow the demons to speak, because they knew Him.

<u>Lk 4:40</u> When the sun was setting, all those who had any that were sick with various diseases brought them to Him; and He laid His hands on every one of them and **healed** them.

<u>Lk 6:17</u> And He came down with them and stood on a level place with a crowd of His disciples and a great multitude of people from all Judea and Jerusalem, and from the seacoast of Tyre and Sidon, who came to hear Him and be **healed** of their diseases,

<u>Acts 28:9</u> So when this was done, the rest of those on the island who had diseases also came and were **healed**.

Dislocation
<u>Heb 12:13</u> and make straight paths for your feet, so that what is lame may not be *dislocated*, but rather be **healed**.

Dysentery

Acts 28:8 And it happened that the father of Publius lay sick of a fever and dysentery. Paul went in to him and prayed, and he laid his hands on him and **healed** him.

Emotional

Ps 147:3 He **heals** the brokenhearted and binds up their wounds.

Isa 61:1, Lk 4:18 The Spirit of the Lord GOD *is* upon Me, because the LORD has anointed Me to preach good tidings to the poor; He has sent Me to **heal** the brokenhearted, to proclaim liberty to the captives, and the opening of the prison to *those who are* bound;

The New Testament contains a number of scriptures that identify the believer's relationship to God. These are identified as the "In Him" verses. They apply to everyone who has been reconciled to God through faith in Jesus Christ. The truth about you is not what you feel or think or believe; it is what God's word says about you.

All who have received Him as their personal Lord and Savior have been born again by the Spirit and have become a new creation in Christ Jesus. 2 Cor. 5:17 "Therefore, if anyone (is) in Christ, (he is) a new creation; old things have passed away; behold, all things have become new." The reality of this truth must be appropriated by faith if the believer is to live a victorious Christian life. ("In Him" verses are not presented here.)

Epilepsy

<u>Mt 4:24</u> Then His fame went throughout all Syria; and they brought to Him all sick people who were afflicted with various diseases and torments, and those who were demon-possessed, epileptics, and paralytics; and He **healed** them.

Fear

<u>Ps 34:4</u> I sought the LORD, and He heard me, and delivered me from all my fears.

<u>Isa 35:4</u> Say to those who are fearful-hearted, "Be strong, do not fear! Behold, your God will come with vengeance, with the recompense of God; He will come and save you."

Feet

<u>Deut 8:4</u> Your garments did not wear out on you, nor did your foot swell these forty years.

<u>Neh 9:21</u> Forty years didst thou sustain them in the wilderness, and they lacked nothing; their clothes did not wear out and their feet did not swell.

<u>Acts 3:7-8</u> And he took him by the right hand and lifted him up, and immediately his feet and ankle bones received strength. 8 So he, leaping up, stood and walked and entered the temple with them--walking, leaping, and praising God.

Fertility

<u>Gen 15:2, 4,</u> And Abram said, "Lord Jehovah, what wilt Thou give me? seeing I go childless,"…4 And behold, the word of Jehovah [came] to him, saying, "This shall not be thine heir, but he that will come forth out of thy body shall be thine heir."

<u>Gen 20:17</u> So Abraham prayed to God, and God **healed** Abimelech, his wife, and his female servants. Then they bore *children*;

<u>Ex 23:26</u> No one shall suffer miscarriage or be barren in your land; I will fulfill the number of your days.

<u>Deut. 7:11-14</u> Therefore you shall keep the commandment, the statutes, and the judgments which I command you today, to observe them. 12 Then it shall come to pass, because you listen to these judgments, and keep and do them, that the LORD your God will keep with you the covenant and the mercy which He swore to your fathers. 13 And He will love you and bless you and multiply you; He will also bless the fruit of your womb and the fruit of your land,… 14 You shall be blessed above all peoples; there shall not be a male or female barren among you or among your livestock.

Fever

<u>Mk 1:30-31</u> But Simon's wife's mother lay sick with a fever, and they told Him about her at once. 31 So He came and took her by the hand and lifted her up, and immediately the fever left her. And she served them.

Acts 28:8 And it happened that the father of Publius lay sick of a fever and dysentery. Paul went in to him and prayed, and he laid his hands on him and **healed** him.

Forgiveness
(Offenses can leave emotional and spiritual wounds)

Neh 1:6-9 Please let Your ear be attentive and Your eyes open, that You may hear the prayer of Your servant which I pray before You now, day and night, for the children of Israel Your servants, and confess the sins of the children of Israel which we have sinned against You. Both my father's house and I have sinned. 7 We have acted very corruptly against You, and have not kept the commandments, the statutes, nor the ordinances which You commanded Your servant Moses. 8 Remember, I pray, the word that You commanded Your servant Moses, saying, 'If you are unfaithful, I will scatter you among the nations; 9 but if you return to Me, and keep My commandments and do them, though some of you were cast out to the farthest part of the heavens, yet I will gather them from there, and bring them to the place which I have chosen as a dwelling for My name.' 10 Now these are Your servants and Your people, whom You have redeemed by Your great power, and by Your strong hand.

Ps 32:5 I acknowledged my sin to You, and my iniquity I have not hidden. I said, "I will confess my transgressions to the LORD," And You forgave the iniquity of my sin. Selah

Ps 103:3-4 Who forgives all your iniquities, Who **heals** all your diseases, 4 Who redeems your life from destruction, Who crowns you with loving kindness and tender mercies,

<u>Isa 1:18</u> "Come now, and let us reason together," Says the LORD, "Though your sins are like scarlet, they shall be as white as snow; Though they are red like crimson, They shall be as wool."

<u>Mt 9:2-7</u> Then behold, they brought to Him a paralytic lying on a bed. When Jesus saw their faith, He said to the paralytic, "Son, be of good cheer; your sins are forgiven you." 3 And at once some of the scribes said within themselves, "This Man blasphemes!" 4 But Jesus, knowing their thoughts, said, "Why do you think evil in your hearts? 5 For which is easier, to say, 'Your sins are forgiven you,' or to say, 'Arise and walk'? 6 But that you may know that the Son of Man has power on earth to forgive sins" --then He said to the paralytic, "Arise, take up your bed, and go to your house." 7 And he arose and departed to his house. 8 Now when the multitudes saw it, they marveled and glorified God, who had given such power to men.

<u>Mk 11:25-26</u> And whenever you stand praying, if you have anything against anyone, forgive him, that your Father in heaven may also forgive you your trespasses. 26 But if you do not forgive, neither will your Father in heaven forgive your trespasses.

<u>I Jn 1:8-10</u> If we say that we have no sin, we deceive ourselves, and the truth is not in us. 9 If we confess our sins, He is faithful and just to forgive us our sins and to cleanse us from all unrighteousness. 10 If we say that we have not sinned, we make Him a liar, and His word is not in us.

General

<u>Deut 32:39</u> Now see that I, *even I, am* He, and *there is* no God besides Me; I kill and I make alive; I wound and I **heal**; nor *is there any* who can deliver from My hand.

<u>Num 12:13</u> So Moses cried out to the LORD, saying, "Please **heal** her, O God, I pray!"

<u>Ps 30:2</u> O LORD my God, I cried out to You, and You **healed** me.

<u>Ps 38</u>

<u>Ps 103:3-4</u> Who forgives all your iniquities, Who heals all your diseases, 4 Who redeems your life from destruction, Who crowns you with loving kindness and tender mercies,

<u>Ps 107:20</u> He sent His word and **healed** them, and delivered them from their destructions.

<u>Pr 3:7-8</u> Do not be wise in your own eyes; Fear the LORD and depart from evil. 8 It will be health to your flesh, and strength to your bones.

<u>Pr 4:22</u> For they *are* life to those who find them, and **health** to all their flesh.

<u>Isa 53:4, 5,</u> Surely He has borne our griefs and carried our sorrows; yet we esteemed Him stricken, smitten by God, and afflicted. But He *was* wounded for our transgressions, *He was* bruised for our iniquities; The chastisement for our peace *was* upon Him, and by His stripes we are **healed**.

Isa 57:18-19 I have seen his ways, and will **heal** him; I will also lead him, and restore comforts to him and to his mourners. 19 I create the fruit of the lips: "Peace, peace to him who is far off and to him who is near," says the LORD, "And I will **heal** him."

Isa 58:8, 9, Then your light shall break forth like the morning, Your **healing** shall spring forth speedily, and your righteousness shall go before you; The glory of the LORD shall be your rear guard. Then you shall call, and the LORD will answer; You shall cry, and He will say, 'Here I am.' If you take away the yoke from your midst, The pointing of the finger, and speaking wickedness,

Jer 17:14 **Heal** me, O LORD, and I shall be **healed**; Save me, and I shall be saved, for You *are* my praise.

Jer 30:17 For I will restore health to you and **heal** you of your wounds, says the LORD.

Jer 33:6 Behold, I will bring **health** and **healing**; I will **heal** them and reveal to them the abundance of peace and truth.

Mal 4:2 But to you who fear My name, the Sun of Righteousness shall arise with **healing** in His wings; and you shall go out and grow fat like stall-fed calves.

Mt 8:7,8,13 And Jesus said to him, "I will come and **heal** him." 8 The centurion answered and said, "Lord, I am not worthy that You should come under my roof. But only speak a word, and my servant will be **healed**." 13 Then Jesus said to the centurion, "Go your way; and as you have believed, *so* let it be done for you." And his servant was **healed** that same hour.

<u>Mt 8:16</u> When evening had come, they brought to Him many who were demon-possessed. And He cast out the spirits with a word, and **healed** all who were sick,

<u>Mt 19:2</u> And great multitudes followed Him, and He **healed** them there.

<u>Lk 5:17</u> Now it happened on a certain day, as He was teaching, that there were Pharisees and teachers of the law sitting by, who had come out of every town of Galilee, Judea, and Jerusalem. And the power of the Lord was *present* to **heal** them.

<u>Lk 6:19</u> And the whole multitude sought to touch Him, for power went out from Him and **healed** *them* all.

<u>Lk 8:48</u> And He said to her, "Daughter, be of good cheer; your faith has made you well. Go in peace."

<u>Lk 9:6</u> So they departed and went through the towns, preaching the gospel and **healing** everywhere.

<u>Lk 9:11</u> But when the multitudes knew *it*, they followed Him; and He received them and spoke to them about the kingdom of God, and **healed** those who had need of **healing**.

<u>Acts 4:30</u> by stretching out Your hand to **heal**, and that signs and wonders may be done through the name of Your holy Servant Jesus.

<u>Acts 5:16</u> Also a multitude gathered from the surrounding cities to Jerusalem, bringing sick people and those who were tormented by unclean spirits, and they were all **healed**.

Acts 28:27 For the hearts of this people have grown dull. Their ears are hard of hearing, and their eyes they have closed, lest they should see with their eyes and hear with their ears, lest they should understand with their hearts and turn, so that I should **heal** them.

1 Thes 5:23 Now may the God of peace Himself sanctify you completely; and may your whole spirit, soul, and body be preserved blameless at the coming of our Lord Jesus Christ.

Jas 5:16 Confess your trespasses to one another, and pray for one another, that you may be **healed**. The effective, fervent prayer of a righteous man avails much.

1 Pet 2:24 and He Himself bore our sins in His body on the cross, that we might die to sin and live to righteousness; for by His wounds you were **healed**. (NASB)

1Pet 2:24 who Himself bore our sins in His own body on the tree, that we, having died to sins, might live for righteousness--by whose stripes you were **healed**.

Hands

I Ki 13:6 Then the king answered and said to the man of God, "Please entreat the favor of the LORD your God, and pray for me, that my hand may be restored to me." So the man of God entreated the LORD, and the king's hand was restored to him, and became as before.

Isa 35:3-4 Strengthen the weak hands, and make firm the feeble knees. 4 Say to those who are fearful-hearted, "Be strong, do not fear! Behold, your God will come with vengeance, with the recompense of God; He will come and save you."

Heb 12:12-13 Therefore strengthen the hands which hang down, and the feeble knees, 13 and make straight paths for your feet, so that what is lame may not be dislocated, but rather be **healed**.

Headaches

2 Ki 4:19, 32-35 And he said to his father, "My head, my head!" So he said to a servant, "Carry him to his mother." 32 When Elisha came into the house, there was the child, lying dead on his bed. 33 He went in therefore, shut the door behind the two of them, and prayed to the LORD. 34 And he went up and lay on the child, and put his mouth on his mouth, his eyes on his eyes, and his hands on his hands; and he stretched himself out on the child, and the flesh of the child became warm. 35 He returned and walked back and forth in the house, and again went up and stretched himself out on him; then the child sneezed seven times, and the child opened his eyes.

Health

Pr 3:7-8 Do not be wise in your own eyes; Fear the LORD and depart from evil. 8 It will be health to your flesh, and strength to your bones.

<u>Pr 4:20-22</u> My son, give attention to my words; Incline your ear to my sayings. 21 Do not let them depart from your eyes; Keep them in the midst of your heart; 22 For they are life to those who find them, and health to all their flesh.

Heart *(See Ministry Helps, Heart Disease--Prayer & Counsel for)*
<u>Ps 147:3</u> He **heals** the brokenhearted And binds up their wounds.

<u>Isa 35:4</u> Say to those who are fearful-hearted, "Be strong, do not fear! Behold, your God will come with vengeance, with the recompense of God; He will come and save you."

<u>Isa 61:1, Lk 4:18</u> The Spirit of the Lord GOD *is* upon Me, because the LORD has anointed Me to preach good tidings to the poor; He has sent Me to **heal** the brokenhearted, to proclaim liberty to the captives, and the opening of the prison to *those who are* bound;

<u>Acts 28:27</u> For the hearts of this people have grown dull. Their ears are hard of hearing, and their eyes they have closed, lest they should see with their eyes and hear with their ears, lest they should understand with their hearts and turn, so that I should heal them.

Hemorrhage

<u>Mk 5:25-34,</u> And a woman who had had a hemorrhage for twelve years, and had endured much at the hands of many physicians, and had spent all that she had and was not helped at all, but rather had grown worse, after hearing about Jesus, came up in the crowd behind *Him,* and touched His cloak. For she thought, "If I just touch His garments, I shall get well." And immediately the flow of her blood was dried up; and she felt in her body that she was healed of her affliction. And immediately Jesus, perceiving in Himself that the power *proceeding* from Him had gone forth, turned around in the crowd and said, "Who touched My garments?" And His disciples said to Him, "You see the multitude pressing in on You, and You say, 'Who touched Me?'" And He looked around to see the woman who had done this. But the woman fearing and trembling, aware of what had happened to her, came and fell down before Him, and told Him the whole truth. And He said to her, "Daughter, your faith has made you well; go in peace, and be **healed** of your affliction." (NASB)

<u>Lk 8:43,47</u> Now a woman, having a flow of blood for twelve years, who had spent all her livelihood on physicians and could not be **healed** by any,47 Now when the woman saw that she was not hidden, she came trembling; and falling down before Him, she declared to Him in the presence of all the people the reason she had touched Him and how she was **healed** immediately.

Infirmities

<u>Mt 4:23</u> And Jesus went about all Galilee, teaching in their synagogues, preaching the gospel of the kingdom, and **healing** all kinds of sickness and all kinds of disease among the people.

<u>Mt 4:24</u> Then His fame went throughout all Syria; and they brought to Him all sick people who were afflicted with various diseases and torments, and those who were demon-possessed, epileptics, and paralytics; and He **healed** them.

<u>Mt 8:16-17</u> When evening had come, they brought to Him many who were demon-possessed. And He cast out the spirits with a word, and healed all who were sick, 17 that it might be fulfilled which was spoken by Isaiah the prophet, saying: "He Himself took our infirmities and bore our sicknesses."

<u>Mt 9:35</u> Then Jesus went about all the cities and villages, teaching in their synagogues, preaching the gospel of the kingdom, and **healing** every sickness and every disease among the people.

<u>Mt 10:1</u> And when He had called His twelve disciples to *Him*, He gave them power *over* unclean spirits, to cast them out, and to **heal** all kinds of sickness and all kinds of disease.

<u>Mt 10:8</u> **Heal** the sick, cleanse the lepers, raise the dead, cast out demons. Freely you have received, freely give.

<u>Mt 14:14</u> And when Jesus went out He saw a great multitude; and He was moved with compassion for them, and **healed** their sick.

<u>Mk 1:34</u> Then He **healed** many who were sick with various diseases, and cast out many demons; and He did not allow the demons to speak, because they knew Him.

<u>Mk 3:15</u> and to have power to **heal** sicknesses and to cast out demons:

Mk 6:13 And they cast out many demons, and anointed with oil many who were sick, and **healed** *them.*

Lk 4:40 When the sun was setting, all those who had any that were sick with various diseases brought them to Him; and He laid His hands on every one of them and **healed** them.

Lk 5:15 However, the report went around concerning Him all the more; and great multitudes came together to hear, and to be **healed** by Him of their infirmities.

Lk 7:3,7,10 So when he heard about Jesus, he sent elders of the Jews to Him, pleading with Him to come and **heal** his servant. 7 "Therefore I did not even think myself worthy to come to You. But say the word, and my servant will be **healed**.10 Then the men who had been sent returned to the house and found the servant **well.**

Lk 8:2 and certain women who had been **healed** of evil spirits and infirmities--Mary called Magdalene, out of whom had come seven demons,

Lk 9:2 He sent them to preach the kingdom of God and to **heal** the sick.

Lk 10:9 And **heal** the sick there, and say to them, 'The kingdom of God has come near to you.'

Acts 5:16 Also a multitude gathered from the surrounding cities to Jerusalem, bringing sick people and those who were tormented by unclean spirits, and they were all **healed**.

Acts 28:9 So when this was done, the rest of those on the island who had diseases also came and were **healed**.

Jas 5:13-16, Is anyone among you suffering? Let him pray. Is anyone cheerful? Let him sing psalms. Is anyone among you sick? Let him call for the elders of the church, and let them pray over him, anointing him with oil in the name of the Lord. And the prayer of faith will save the sick, and the Lord will raise him up. And if he has committed sins, he will be forgiven. Confess *your* trespasses to one another, and pray for one another, that you may be **healed**. The effective, fervent prayer of a righteous man avails much."

Inflammation
Ps 38:5-8,15 My wounds are foul and festering because of my foolishness. 6 I am troubled, I am bowed down greatly; I go mourning all the day long. 7 For my loins are full of inflammation, and there is no soundness in my flesh. 8 I am feeble and severely broken; I groan because of the turmoil of my heart. 15 For in You, O LORD, I hope; You will hear, O Lord my God.

Invalid
Jn 5:13 But the one who was **healed** did not know who it was, for Jesus had withdrawn, a multitude being in that place.

Knees

Isa 35:3-4 Strengthen the weak hands, and make firm the feeble knees. 4 Say to those who are fearful-hearted, "Be strong, do not fear! Behold, your God will come with vengeance, with the recompense of God; He will come and save you."

Heb 12:12-13 Therefore strengthen the hands which hang down, and the feeble knees, 13 and make straight paths for your feet, so that what is lame may not be dislocated, but rather be **healed**.

Lame

Zeph 3:19 Behold, at that time I will deal with all who afflict you; I will save the lame, and gather those who were driven out; I will appoint them for praise and fame in every land where they were put to shame.

Mt 15:30 Then great multitudes came to Him, having with them the lame, blind, mute, maimed, and many others; and they laid them down at Jesus' feet, and He **healed** them.

Mt 21:14 Then the blind and the lame came to Him in the temple, and He **healed** them.

Acts 3:11 Now as the lame man who was **healed** held on to Peter and John, all the people ran together to them in the porch which is called Solomon's, greatly amazed.

Acts 9:34 And Peter said to him, "Aeneas, Jesus the Christ **heals** you. Arise and make your bed." Then he arose immediately.

<u>Acts 14:8</u> there sat a man crippled in his feet, who was lame from birth and had never walked.

<u>Acts 14:9</u> *This* man heard Paul speaking. Paul, observing him intently and seeing that he had faith to be **healed**,

<u>Heb 12:13</u> and make straight paths for your feet, so that what is lame may not be *dislocated*, but rather be **healed**.

Leprosy

<u>Nu 12:13</u> So Moses cried out to the LORD, saying, "Please **heal** her, O God, I pray!"

<u>2Ki 5:6-7, 11</u> Then he brought the letter to the king of Israel, which said, "Now be advised, when this letter comes to you, that I have sent Naaman my servant to you, that you may **heal** him of his leprosy." 7 And it happened, when the king of Israel read the letter, that he tore his clothes and said, "*Am* I God, to kill and make alive, that this man sends a man to me to **heal** him of his leprosy? Therefore please consider, and see how he seeks a quarrel with me." 11 But Naaman became furious, and went away and said, "Indeed, I said to myself, 'He will surely come out *to me*, and stand and call on the name of the LORD his God, and wave his hand over the place, and **heal** the leprosy.'

<u>Mt 8:2,3</u> And behold, a leper came and worshiped Him, saying, "Lord, if You are willing, You can make me clean." 3 Then Jesus put out His hand and touched him, saying, "I am willing; be cleansed." Immediately his leprosy was cleansed.

Mt 10:8 **Heal** the sick, cleanse the lepers, raise the dead, cast out demons. Freely you have received, freely give.

Life and Extended Life

Ex 23:25-26 So you shall serve the LORD your God, and He will bless your bread and your water. And I will take sickness away from the midst of you. 26 No one shall suffer miscarriage or be barren in your land; I will fulfill the number of your days.

Deut 30:6 And the LORD your God will circumcise your heart and the heart of your descendants, to love the LORD your God with all your heart and with all your soul, that you may live.

Ruth 4:15 And may he be to you a restorer of life and a nourisher of your old age; for your daughter-in-law, who loves you, who is better to you than seven sons, has borne him.

2Ki 4:19, 32-35 And he said to his father, "My head, my head!" So he said to a servant, "Carry him to his mother." When Elisha came into the house, there was the child, lying dead on his bed. 33 He went in therefore, shut the door behind the two of them, and prayed to the LORD. 34 And he went up and lay on the child, and put his mouth on his mouth, his eyes on his eyes, and his hands on his hands; and he stretched himself out on the child, and the flesh of the child became warm. 35 He returned and walked back and forth in the house, and again went up and stretched himself out on him; then the child sneezed seven times, and the child opened his eyes.

<u>Ps 21:4</u> He asked life from You, and You gave it to him. Length of days forever and ever.

<u>Ps 41:2,3</u> Jehovah will preserve him, and keep him alive. 3 The LORD will strengthen him on his bed of illness; You will sustain him on his sickbed.

<u>Ps 56:13</u> For You have delivered my soul from death. Have You not kept my feet from falling, that I may walk before God in the light of the living?

<u>Ps 72:13</u> He will spare the poor and needy, and will save the souls of the needy.

<u>Ps 79:11</u> Let the groaning of the prisoner come before You; According to the greatness of Your power preserve those who are appointed to die;

<u>Ps 102:23-24</u> He weakened my strength in the way; He shortened my days. 24 I said, "O my God, do not take me away in the midst of my days; Your years are throughout all generations

<u>Ps 103:3-5</u> Who forgives all your iniquities, Who **heals** all your diseases, 4 Who redeems your life from the Pit, Who crowns you with steadfast love and mercy, 5 Who satisfies you with good as long as you live so that your youth is renewed like the eagle's.

<u>Ps 107:18-20</u> Their soul abhorred all manner of food, and they drew near to the gates of death. 19 Then they cried out to the LORD in their trouble, and He saved them out of their distresses. 20 He sent His word and **healed** them, and delivered them from their destructions.

Ps 116:1-9 I love the LORD, because He has heard My voice and my supplications. 2 Because He has inclined His ear to me, therefore I will call upon Him as long as I live. 3 The pains of death surrounded me, and the pangs of Sheol laid hold of me; I found trouble and sorrow. 4 Then I called upon the name of the LORD: "O LORD, I implore You, deliver my soul!" 5 Gracious is the LORD, and righteous; Yes, our God is merciful. 6 The LORD preserves the simple; I was brought low, and He saved me. 7 Return to your rest, O my soul, for the LORD has dealt bountifully with you. 8 For You have delivered my soul from death, my eyes from tears, and my feet from falling. 9 I will walk before the LORD In the land of the living.

Ps 118:17-18 I shall not die, but live, and declare the works of the LORD. 18 The LORD has chastened me severely, but He has not given me over to death.

Ps 119:116-7,154 Uphold me according to Your word, that I may live; and do not let me be ashamed of my hope. 117 Hold me up, and I shall be safe, and I shall observe Your statutes continually. 154 Plead my cause and redeem me; Revive me according to Your word.

Pr 3:21-23 My son, let them not depart from your eyes. Keep sound wisdom and discretion; 22 So they will be life to your soul and grace to your neck. 23 Then you will walk safely in your way, and your foot will not stumble.

Pr 4:20-22 My son, give attention to My words; Incline your ear to My sayings. 21 Do not let them depart from your eyes; Keep them in the midst of your heart; 22 For they are life to those who find them, and health to all their flesh.

Pr 8:35 For whoever finds Me finds life, and obtains favor from the LORD.

Prov 18:21 Death and life are in the power of the tongue, and those who love it will eat its fruit.

Isa 38:5 'Thus says the LORD, the God of David your father: "I have heard your prayer, I have seen your tears; surely I will add to your days fifteen years.

Jn 11:4 When Jesus heard that, He said, "This sickness is not unto death, but for the glory of God, that the Son of God may be glorified through it."

Rom 8:11 But if the Spirit of Him who raised Jesus from the dead dwells in you, He who raised Christ from the dead will also give life to your mortal bodies through His Spirit who dwells in you.

Maimed

Mt 15:30 Then great multitudes came to Him, having with them the lame, blind, mute, maimed, and many others; and they laid them down at Jesus' feet, and He **healed** them.

Mute

Mt 12:22 Then one was brought to Him who was demon-possessed, blind and mute; and He **healed** him, so that the blind and mute man both spoke and saw.

<u>Mt 15:30</u> Then great multitudes came to Him, having with them the lame, blind, mute, maimed, and many others; and they laid them down at Jesus' feet, and He **healed** them.

<u>Mk 7:37</u> And they were astonished beyond measure, saying, "He has done all things well. He makes both the deaf to hear and the mute to speak."

Old Age
<u>Ruth 4:15</u> And he shall be to thee a restorer of thy life, and a nourisher of thine old age;

<u>Ex 23:26</u> No one shall suffer miscarriage or be barren in your land; I will fulfill the number of your days.

Oppression
<u>Lk 4:18,</u> The Spirit of the LORD *is* upon Me, because He has anointed Me to preach the gospel to the poor; He has sent Me to **heal** the brokenhearted, to proclaim liberty to the captives and recovery of sight to the blind, to set at liberty those who are oppressed;

Pain
<u>Ps 69:29</u> But I am afflicted and in pain; let thy salvation, O God, set me on high! (RSV)

<u>Mt 4:24</u> News about Him spread all over Syria, and people brought to Him all who were ill with various diseases, those suffering severe pain, the demon-possessed, those having seizures, and the paralyzed, and He **healed** them. (NIV)

Paralytics

<u>Mt 8:7,8,13</u> And Jesus said to him, "I will come and **heal** him." 8 The centurion answered and said, "Lord, I am not worthy that You should come under my roof. But only speak a word, and my servant will be **healed.**" 13 Then Jesus said to the centurion, "Go your way; and as you have believed, *so* let it be done for you." And his servant was **healed** that same hour.

<u>Mt 4:24</u> Then His fame went throughout all Syria; and they brought to Him all sick people who were afflicted with various diseases and torments, and those who were demon-possessed, epileptics, and paralytics; and He **healed** them. (RSV)

<u>Mt 9:2, 5-7</u> Then behold, they brought to Him a paralytic lying on a bed. When Jesus saw their faith, He said to the paralytic, "Son, be of good cheer; your sins are forgiven you." 5 For which is easier to say, 'Your sins are forgiven you,' or to say, 'Arise and walk'?" 6 But that you may know that the Son of Man has power on earth to forgive sins --then He said to the paralytic, "Arise, take up your bed, and go to your house."

Poison

<u>Mk 16:18</u> they will take up serpents; and if they drink anything deadly, it will by no means hurt them; they will lay hands on the sick, and they will **recover**."

Resurrection Power

<u>Mt 10:8</u> **Heal** the sick, cleanse the lepers, raise the dead, cast out demons. Freely you have received, freely give.

<u>Mk 5:39 & 41</u> When He came in, He said to them, "Why make this commotion and weep? The child is not dead, but sleeping." 41 Then He took the child by the hand, and said to her, "Talitha, cumi," which is translated, "Little girl, I say to you, arise."

<u>Jn 11:23, 41-44</u> Jesus said to her, "Your brother will rise again." 41 Then they took away the stone from the place where the dead man was lying. And Jesus lifted up His eyes and said, "Father, I thank You that You have heard Me. 42 And I know that You always hear Me, but because of the people who are standing by I said this, that they may believe that You sent Me." 43 Now when He had said these things, He cried with a loud voice, "Lazarus, come forth!" 44 And he who had died came out bound hand and foot with grave clothes, and his face was wrapped with a cloth. Jesus said to them, "Loose him, and let him go."

Revive

Hos 6:1-2 Come, and let us return to the LORD; for He has torn, but He will **heal** us; He has stricken, but He will bind us up. 2 After two days He will revive us; On the third day He will raise us up, that we may live in His sight.

Save

Jn 12:47 And if anyone hears My words and does not believe, I do not judge him; for I did not come to judge the world but to save the world.

Seizures

Mt 4:24 News about Him spread all over Syria, and people brought to Him all who were ill with various diseases, those suffering severe pain, the demon-possessed, those having seizures, and the paralyzed, and He **healed** them. (NIV)

Sickness

Ex 23:25 So you shall serve the LORD your God, and He will bless your bread and your water. And I will take sickness away from the midst of you.

Deut. 7:11,12,15 Therefore you shall keep the commandment, the statutes, and the judgments which I command you today, to observe them. 12 Then it shall come to pass, because you listen to these judgments, and keep and do them, that the LORD your God will keep with you the covenant and the mercy which He swore to your fathers. 15 And the LORD will take away from you all sickness, and will afflict you with none of the terrible diseases of Egypt which you have known, but will lay them on all those who hate you.

Ps 41:3 The LORD will strengthen him on his bed of illness; You will sustain him on his sickbed.

Mt 4:23-24 And Jesus went about all Galilee, teaching in their synagogues, preaching the gospel of the kingdom, and **healing** all kinds of sickness and all kinds of disease among the people. 24 Then His fame went throughout all Syria; and they brought to Him all sick people who were afflicted with various diseases and torments, and those who were demon-possessed, epileptics, and paralytics; and He **healed** them.

Mt 9:35 Then Jesus went about all the cities and villages, teaching in their synagogues, preaching the gospel of the kingdom, and **healing** every sickness and every disease among the people.

Mt 10:1 And when He had called His twelve disciples to Him, He gave them power *over* unclean spirits, to cast them out, and to **heal** all kinds of sickness and all kinds of disease.

Mt 14:14 And when Jesus went out He saw a great multitude; and He was moved with compassion for them, and **healed** their sick.

<u>Mk 1:34</u> Then He **healed** many who were sick with various diseases, and cast out many demons; and He did not allow the demons to speak, because they knew Him.

<u>Mk 3:15</u> and to have power to **heal** sicknesses and to cast out demons:

<u>Mk 6:13</u> And they cast out many demons, and anointed with oil many who were sick, and **healed** *them.*

<u>Lk 4:40</u> When the sun was setting, all those who had any that were sick with various diseases brought them to Him; and He laid His hands on every one of them and **healed** them.

<u>Lk 5:15</u> However, the report went around concerning Him all the more; and great multitudes came together to hear, and to be **healed** by Him of their infirmities.

<u>Lk 7:3,7,10</u> So when he heard about Jesus, he sent elders of the Jews to Him, pleading with Him to come and **heal** his servant. 7 "Therefore I did not even think myself worthy to come to You. But say the word, and my servant will be **healed**." 10 Then the men who had been sent returned to the house and found the servant **well**.

<u>Lk 9:2</u> He sent them to preach the kingdom of God and to **heal** the sick.

<u>Lk 10:9</u> And **heal** the sick there, and say to them, "The kingdom of God has come near to you."

<u>Acts 5:16</u> Also a multitude gathered from the surrounding cities to Jerusalem, bringing sick people and those who were tormented by unclean spirits, and they were all **healed**.

<u>Jas 5:13-16,</u> Is anyone among you suffering? Let him pray. Is anyone cheerful? Let him sing psalms. Is anyone among you sick? Let him call for the elders of the church, and let them pray over him, anointing him with oil in the name of the Lord. And the prayer of faith will save the sick, and the Lord will raise him up. And if he has committed sins, he will be forgiven. Confess *your* trespasses to one another, and pray for one another, that you may be **healed**. The effective, fervent prayer of a righteous man avails much.

Sleep

<u>Job 11:18-19</u> And you will have confidence, because there is hope; you will be protected and take your rest in safety. 19 You will lie down, and none will make you afraid; many will entreat your favor. (RSV)

<u>Pr 3:24</u> When you lie down, you will not be afraid; Yes, you will lie down and your sleep will be sweet.

Snake Bite

<u>Mk 16:18</u> they will take up serpents; and if they drink anything deadly, it will by no means hurt them; they will lay hands on the sick, and they will recover.

Sorrow

Ex 3:7-8 And Jehovah said, "I have surely seen the affliction of my people…and have heard their cry…for I know their sorrows; 8 So I have come down to deliver them." (ASV)

Ps 69:29 But I am poor and sorrowful; Let Your salvation, O God, set me up on high.

Ps 116:1-9 I love the LORD, because He has heard My voice and my supplications. 2 Because He has inclined His ear to me, therefore I will call upon Him as long as I live. 3 The pains of death surrounded me, and the pangs of Sheol laid hold of me; I found trouble and sorrow. 4 Then I called upon the name of the LORD: "O LORD, I implore You, deliver my soul!" 5 Gracious is the LORD, and righteous; Yes, our God is merciful. 6 The LORD preserves the simple; I was brought low, and He saved me. 7 Return to your rest, O my soul, for the LORD has dealt bountifully with you. 8 For You have delivered my soul from death, my eyes from tears, and my feet from falling. 9 I will walk before the LORD In the land of the living.

Isa 14:3 It shall come to pass in the day the LORD gives you rest from your sorrow, and from your fear and the hard bondage in which you were made to serve,

Isa 51:11 So the ransomed of the LORD shall return, and come to Zion with singing, with everlasting joy on their heads. They shall obtain joy and gladness; Sorrow and sighing shall flee away.

Isa 53:4 Surely He has borne our griefs and carried our sorrows; Yet we esteemed Him stricken, Smitten by God, and afflicted.

Suffering

<u>Ps 119:49-50</u> Remember Your word to Your servant, for You have given me hope. My comfort in my suffering is this: Your promise preserves my life. (NIV)

<u>Mk 5:34</u> He said to her, "Daughter, your faith has **healed** you. Go in peace and be freed from your suffering." (NIV)

<u>Heb 5:7-8</u> Who, in the days of His flesh, when He had offered up prayers and supplications, with vehement cries and tears to Him who was able to save Him from death, and was heard because of His godly fear, 8 though He was a Son, yet He learned obedience by the things which He suffered.

Walk

<u>Mt 9:2-7</u> Then behold, they brought to Him a paralytic lying on a bed. When Jesus saw their faith, He said to the paralytic, "Son, be of good cheer; your sins are forgiven you." 3 And at once some of the scribes said within themselves, "This Man blasphemes!" 4 But Jesus, knowing their thoughts, said, "Why do you think evil in your hearts? 5 For which is easier, to say, 'Your sins are forgiven you,' or to say, 'Arise and walk'?" 6 "But that you may know that the Son of Man has power on earth to forgive sins" --then He said to the paralytic, "Arise, take up your bed, and go to your house." 7 And he arose and departed to his house.

<u>Acts 3:6-8</u> Then Peter said, "Silver and gold I do not have, but what I do have I give you: In the name of Jesus Christ of Nazareth, rise up and walk." 7 And he took him by the right hand and

lifted him up, and immediately his feet and ankle bones received strength. 8 So he, leaping up, stood and walked and entered the temple with them—walking, leaping, and praising God.

Wounds

Ps 147:3 He **heals** the brokenhearted and binds up their wounds.

Isa 30:26 ... In the day that the LORD binds up the bruise of His people and **heals** the stroke of their wound.

Jer 30:17 "For I will restore health to you and **heal** you of your wounds," says the LORD.

Hos 6:1,2 Come, and let us return to the LORD; For He has torn, but He will **heal** us; He has stricken, but He will bind us up. 2 After two days He will revive us; On the third day He will raise us up, that we may live in His sight.

Lk 22:51 But Jesus answered and said, "Permit even this." And He touched his ear and **healed** him.

MINISTRY HELPS

Authority over Satan

Mt 10:1 And when He had called His twelve disciples to Him, He gave them power over unclean spirits, to cast them out, and to **heal** all kinds of sickness and all kinds of disease.

Lk 10:18-19 And He said to them, "I saw Satan fall like lightning from heaven. 19 Behold, I give you the authority to trample on serpents and scorpions, and over all the power of the enemy, and nothing shall by any means hurt you."

Jn 12:31 Now is the judgment of this world; now the ruler of this world will be cast out.

Acts 10:38 how God anointed Jesus of Nazareth with the Holy Spirit and with power, who went about doing good and **healing** all who were oppressed by the devil, for God was with Him.

Acts 26:17-18 I will deliver you from the Jewish people, as well as from the Gentiles, to whom I now send you, 18 to open their eyes, in order to turn them from darkness to light, and from the power of Satan to God, that they may receive forgiveness of sins and an inheritance among those who are sanctified by faith in Me.

Commanded and Empowered to Heal

Mt 10:1,7,8 And when He had called His twelve disciples to Him, He gave them power over unclean spirits, to cast them out, and to **heal** all kinds of sickness and all kinds of disease. "And as you go, preach, saying, 'The kingdom of heaven is at hand. 8

Heal the sick, cleanse the lepers, raise the dead, cast out demons. Freely you have received, freely give."

Lk 9:1,2,6 Then He called His twelve disciples together and gave them power and authority over all demons, and to cure diseases. 2 He sent them to preach the kingdom of God and to **heal** the sick. 6 So they departed and went through the towns, preaching the gospel and **healing** everywhere.

Lk 10:1,9 After these things the Lord appointed seventy others also, and sent them two by two before His face into every city and place where He Himself was about to go.9 "And **heal** the sick there, and say to them, 'The kingdom of God has come near to you.'"

Acts 3:6-8 Then Peter said, "Silver and gold I do not have, but what I do have I give you: In the name of Jesus Christ of Nazareth, rise up and walk." 7 And he took him by the right hand and lifted him up, and immediately his feet and ankle bones received strength. 8 So he, leaping up, stood and walked and entered the temple with them—walking, leaping, and praising God.

Comfort During Suffering

Ps 119:50 This is my comfort in my affliction, for Your word has given me life.

Isa 53:4-5 Surely He has borne our griefs and carried our sorrows; Yet we esteemed Him stricken, smitten by God, and afflicted. 5 But He was wounded for our transgressions, He was bruised for our iniquities; The chastisement for our peace was upon Him, and by His stripes we are healed. "Prayer for the Sick" from page 177-178 and delete from page 177-178.

For the Sick

Dear Father, Today we come boldly before Your throne of grace at Your invitation. You have promised that where two or more are gathered, there You will be in the midst of them. So we come today in agreement, asking for Your presence and blessing. Father, our desire is for the healing of _____. We know that because of Jesus suffering there was victory at the cross for us. As we come to You asking forgiveness of our sins, we claim that victory and accept the gift of forgiveness. Lord, there was another victory at the cross. You said that by Your stripes we are healed. We walk in that promise as well; knowing and understanding that healing is not always cure; but that it is the deepest healing of our hearts unto salvation. We thank You that You have a plan and purpose for _____ life. We pray that Your destiny for him/her will be fulfilled. We ask that You would open the windows of heaven and pour out Your grace and mercy over _____ and his/her family as they walk through this health crises/medical challenge. Comfort their hearts and fill them with peace; reminding them that every detail of their life matters to You. In Jesus name, Amen

Death—Supportive Readings at Time of

Ps 23 The LORD is my shepherd; I shall not want. 2 He makes me to lie down in green pastures; He leads me beside the still waters. 3 He restores my soul; He leads me in the paths of righteousness for His name's sake. 4 Yea, though I walk through the valley of the shadow of death, I will fear no evil; For You are with me; Your rod and Your staff, they comfort me. 5 You prepare a table before me in the presence of my enemies; You anoint my head with oil; my cup runs over. 6 Surely goodness and mercy shall follow me all the days of my life; and I will dwell in the house of the LORD forever. Ps 73:24-26 Thou dost guide me with thy counsel, and afterward thou wilt receive me to glory. 25 Whom have I in heaven but thee? And there is nothing upon earth that I desire besides thee. 26 My flesh and my heart may fail, but God is the strength of my heart and my portion forever. (RSV)

Hos 13:14 I will ransom them from the power of the grave; I will redeem them from death. O Death, I will be your plagues! O Grave, I will be your destruction! Pity is hidden from My eyes.

Jn 3:14-16,27 "And as Moses lifted up the serpent in the wilderness, even so must the Son of Man be lifted up, 15 "that whoever believes in Him should not perish but have eternal life. 16 For God so loved the world that He gave His only begotten Son, that whoever believes in Him should not perish but have everlasting life." 27 "Peace I leave with you, My peace I give to you; not as the world gives do I give to you. Let not your heart be troubled, neither let it be afraid."

Jn 14:1-3 "Let not your heart be troubled; you believe in God, believe also in Me. 2 In My Father's house are many mansions; if it were not so, I would have told you. I go to prepare a place for you. 3 And if I go and prepare a place for you, I will come again and receive you to Myself; that where I am, there you may be also."

<u>Rm 8:35-39</u> Who shall separate us from the love of Christ? Shall tribulation, or distress, or persecution, or famine, or nakedness, or peril, or sword? 36 As it is written: "For Your sake we are killed all day long; We are accounted as sheep for the slaughter." 37 Yet in all these things we are more than conquerors through Him who loved us. 38 For I am persuaded that neither death nor life, nor angels nor principalities nor powers, nor things present nor things to come, 39 nor height nor depth, nor any other created thing, shall be able to separate us from the love of God which is in Christ Jesus our Lord.

<u>2 Cor 4:7-18</u> But we have this treasure in earthen vessels, that the excellence of the power may be of God and not of us. 8 We are hard pressed on every side, yet not crushed; we are perplexed, but not in despair; 9 persecuted, but not forsaken; struck down, but not destroyed-- 10 always carrying about in the body the dying of the Lord Jesus, that the life of Jesus also may be manifested in our body. 11 For we who live are always delivered to death for Jesus' sake, that the life of Jesus also may be manifested in our mortal flesh. 12 So then death is working in us, but life in you. 13 And since we have the same spirit of faith, according to what is written, "I believed and therefore I spoke," we also believe and therefore speak, 14 knowing that He who raised up the Lord Jesus will also raise us up with Jesus, and will present us with you. 15 For all things are for your sakes, that grace, having spread through the many, may cause thanksgiving to abound to the glory of God. 16 Therefore we do not lose heart. Even though our outward man is perishing, yet the inward man is being renewed day by day. 17 For our light affliction, which is but for a moment, is working for us a far more exceeding and eternal weight of glory; 18 while we do not look at the things which are seen, but at the things which

are not seen. For the things which are seen are temporary, but the things which are not seen are eternal.

I Thes 4:14-18 For if we believe that Jesus died and rose again, even so God will bring with Him those who sleep in Jesus. 15 For this we say to you by the word of the Lord, that we who are alive and remain until the coming of the Lord will by no means precede those who are asleep. 16 For the Lord Himself will descend from heaven with a shout, with the voice of an archangel, and with the trumpet of God. And the dead in Christ will rise first. 17 Then we who are alive and remain shall be caught up together with them in the clouds to meet the Lord in the air. And thus we shall always be with the Lord. 18 Therefore comfort one another with these words.

Rev 21:1-5 Now I saw a new heaven and a new earth, for the first heaven and the first earth had passed away. Also there was no more sea. 2 Then I, John, saw the holy city, New Jerusalem, coming down out of heaven from God, prepared as a bride adorned for her husband. 3 And I heard a loud voice from heaven saying, "Behold, the tabernacle of God is with men, and He will dwell with them, and they shall be His people. God Himself will be with them and be their God. 4 And God will wipe away every tear from their eyes; there shall be no more death, nor sorrow, nor crying. There shall be no more pain, for the former things have passed away. 5 Then He who sat on the throne said, "Behold, I make all things new." And He said to me, "Write, for these words are true and faithful."

Infant Death

Ps. 139:14, "For You created my inmost being; You knit me together in my mother's womb. I praise You because I am fearfully and wonderfully made."

Jer 31:15, "Thus says the Lord our God: a voice is heard in Ramah, lamentation and bitter weeping. Rachel weeping for her children; she refuses to be comforted for her children are no more."

2 Cor 1:3a,4 (*adapted*) Blessed be our God who consoles us in our affliction, so that we, by grace may be able to console those who are in any affliction with the consolations with which we ourselves are consoled by God.

Infant Death Prayer

Dear Lord, we do not know why this precious treasure is gone from us. We do not understand why so many of our hopes and dreams have now been dashed. Our hearts cry out to you in pain and question.

Today we recognize the fragility of the gift of life. Our expectations have turned to heartache and disappointment. As our hearts cry out, as our arms are empty, we pray for grace and mercy to help us walk in the power of faith through this trial and keep us close to you. We pray that You will wrap us in Your arms of love and hold us close to Your heart. We pray that Your tears will mingle with ours and that Your comfort will be poured out abundantly. May Your presence and love engulf us. In Jesus blessed name, Amen

Heart Disease--Prayer & Counsel for

1. Break any family (generational) curses and command healing of other body parts affected.

2. Pray for a new heart Ez 36:36,27 "I will give you a new heart and put a new spirit within you; I will take the heart of stone out of your flesh and give you a heart of flesh. 27 I will put My Spirit within you and cause you to walk in My statutes, and you will keep My judgments and do them."

3. Love Mt 22:36-40 "Teacher, which is the great commandment in the law?"37 Jesus said to him, "You shall love the LORD your God with all your heart, with all your soul, and with all your mind. 38 This is the first and great commandment. 39 And the second is like it: You shall love your neighbor as yourself."

4. Look to future Phil 3:13 Brethren, I do not count myself to have apprehended; but one thing I do, forgetting those things which are behind and reaching forward to those things which are ahead,

Help with Finances

Ps 35:27 Let them shout for joy and be glad, who favor my righteous cause; and let them say continually, "Let the LORD be magnified, Who has pleasure in the prosperity of His servant."

Mal 3:10 "Bring the whole tithe into the storehouse, that there may be food in My house. Test Me in this," says the Lord Almighty, "and see if I will not throw open the floodgates of heaven and pour out so much blessing that you will not have room enough for it."

Peace

Ps 29:11 The LORD will give strength to His people; The LORD will bless His people with peace.

Isa 55:12 For you shall go out with joy, and be led out with peace; The mountains and the hills shall break forth into singing before you, and all the trees of the field shall clap their hands.

Isa 57:18-19 I have seen his ways, and will **heal** him; I will also lead him, and restore comforts to him and to his mourners. 19 I create the fruit of the lips: "Peace, peace to him who is far off and to him who is near," Says the LORD, "And I will heal him."

Jn 14:27 "Peace I leave with you, My peace I give to you; not as the world gives do I give to you. Let not your heart be troubled, neither let it be afraid."

Recovery

Ps 34:4-8 I sought the LORD, and He heard me, and delivered me from all my fears. 5 They looked to Him and were radiant, and their faces were not ashamed. 6 This poor man cried out, and the LORD heard him, and saved him out of all his troubles. 7 The angel of the LORD encamps all around those who fear Him, and delivers them. 8 Oh, taste and see that the LORD is good; Blessed is the man who trusts in Him!

Ps 107:1,2,6 Oh, give thanks to the LORD, for He is good! For His mercy endures forever. 2 Let the redeemed of the LORD say so, whom He has redeemed from the hand of the enemy, 6 Then they cried out to the LORD in their trouble, and He delivered them out of their distresses.

Seek God First

2 Chron 16:12 And in the thirty-ninth year of his reign, Asa became diseased in his feet, and his malady was severe; yet in his disease he did not seek the LORD, but the physicians.

Speaking

Pr 18:21 Death and life are in the power of the tongue, and those who love it will eat its fruit.

Ex 4:12, 15 Now therefore, go, and I will be with your mouth and teach you what you shall say. 15 Now you shall speak to him and put the words in his mouth. And I will be with your mouth and with his mouth, and I will teach you what you shall do.

Strength

Ps 29:11 Jehovah will give strength unto his people; Jehovah will bless his people with peace. (ASV)

Surgery(Before)

Ps 56:11 In God I have put my trust; I will not be afraid. What can man do to me?

Ps 91

Ps 103:1-5 Bless the LORD, O my soul; And all that is within me, bless His holy name! 2 Bless the LORD, O my soul, and forget not all His benefits: 3 Who forgives all your iniquities, Who heals all your diseases, 4 Who redeems your life from destruction, Who crowns you with loving kindness and tender mercies, 5 Who satisfies your mouth with good things, so that your youth is renewed like the eagle's.

Isa 43:1-3 But now, thus says the LORD, who created you, O Jacob, and He who formed you, O Israel: "Fear not, for I have redeemed you; I have called you by your name; you are Mine. 2 When you pass through the waters, I will be with you; and through the rivers, they shall not overflow you. When you walk through the fire, you shall not be burned, nor shall the flame scorch you. 3 For I am the LORD your God, the Holy One of Israel, your Savior;

Isa 58:8,9 Then your light shall break forth like the morning, your healing shall spring forth speedily, And your righteousness shall go before you; The glory of the LORD shall be your rear guard. 9 Then you shall call, and the LORD will answer; you shall cry, and He will say, 'Here I am.' "

Prayer For Surgery

Heavenly Father, we come to you today in behalf of _____
who is facing surgery. We ask that you will hand pick the medical staff that will be ministering to his/her needs. We pray that You will work through them with skill and expertise beyond themselves, that they too will know they have been touched by the hand of God. We ask that You will fill the room with ministering angels surrounding _____. *If there is any hallucinating, may he/she hallucinate about the Lord Jesus Christ. We come against the spirit of fear and cover* _____ *with the armor of God that the devil may have no inroads. We ask You to carry his/her pain and suffering/sorrow as You have promised and expedite the healing process. May* _____ *find comfort, courage, and peace in Your presence as he/she trust in You. In Jesus name, Amen*

MINISTRY SERVICES/BLESSINGS/PRAYERS

Anointing and Laying On of Hands

Jas 5:14-15 Is anyone among you sick? Let him call for the elders of the church, and let them pray over him, **anointing him with oil in the name of the Lord.** 15 And the prayer of faith will save the sick, and the Lord will raise him up. And if he has committed sins, he will be forgiven.

Mk 6:13 And they cast out many demons, and **anointed with oil** many who were sick, and healed them. In the last paragraph please put in bold line 2, "**lay hands on**" After this paragraph, please add the three following paragraphs:

Mk 5:23 and begged Him earnestly saying, "My little daughter lies at the point of death. Come and **lay Your hands on** her that she may be **healed**, and she will live."

Mk 16:18 they will take up serpents; and if they drink anything deadly, it will by no means hurt them; they will lay hands on the sick, and they will **recover**."

Lk 4:40 When the sun was setting, all those who had any that were sick with various diseases brought them to Him; and He **laid His hands on** every one of them and **healed** them.

Acts 28:8 And it happened that the father of Publius lay sick of a fever and dysentery. Paul went in to him and prayed, and he **laid his hands on** him and **healed** him.

Baptism

If a dying person desires baptism, you may administer it by pouring water on their forehead or by doing a foot washing ceremony, using the person's name, say, "I now baptize you in the name of the Father, the Son, and the Holy Spirit. Amen

Communion *(See Chapter Pastoral Tools, Section Sacred Symbols of Sacraments/Ordinances)*

Lk 22:14-20 When the hour had come, He sat down, and the twelve apostles with Him. 15 Then He said to them, "With fervent desire I have desired to eat this Passover with you before I suffer; 16 for I say to you, I will no longer eat of it until it is fulfilled in the kingdom of God." 17 Then He took the cup, and gave thanks, and said, "Take this and divide it among yourselves; 18 for I say to you, I will not drink of the fruit of the vine until the kingdom of God comes." 19 And He took bread, gave thanks and broke it, and gave it to them, saying, "This is My body which is given for you; do this in remembrance of Me." 20 Likewise He also took the cup after supper, saying, "This cup is the new covenant in My blood, which is shed for you.

I Cor 11:23-32 For I received from the Lord that which I also delivered to you: that the Lord Jesus on the same night in which He was betrayed took bread; 24 and when He had given thanks, He broke it and said, "Take, eat; this is My body which is broken for you; do this in remembrance of Me." 25 In the same manner He also took the cup after supper, saying, "This cup is the new covenant in My blood. This do, as often as you drink it, in remembrance of Me. 26 For as often as you eat this bread and drink this cup, you proclaim the Lord's death till He comes." 27 Therefore whoever eats this bread or drinks this cup of the Lord in an unworthy manner will be guilty of the body and blood of the Lord. 28 But let a man examine himself, and so let him eat of the bread and drink of the cup. 29 For he who eats and drinks in an unworthy manner eats and drinks judgment to himself, not discerning the Lord's body. 30 For this reason many are weak and sick among you, and many sleep. 31 For if we would judge ourselves, we would not be judged. 32 But when we are judged, we are chastened by the Lord, that we may not be condemned with the world.

BLESSINGS
Childbirth/Child dedication or blessing

Mt 18:1-6 At that time the disciples came to Jesus, saying, "Who then is greatest in the kingdom of heaven?" 2 Then Jesus called a little child to Him, set him in the midst of them, 3 and said, "Assuredly, I say to you, unless you are converted and become as little children, you will by no means enter the kingdom of heaven. 4 Therefore whoever humbles himself as this little child is the greatest in the kingdom of heaven. 5 Whoever receives one little child like this in My name receives Me."

Mk 10:13-16 Then they brought little children to Him, that He might touch them; but the disciples rebuked those who brought them. 14 But when Jesus saw it, He was greatly displeased and said to them, "Let the little children come to Me, and do not forbid them; for of such is the kingdom of God. 15 Assuredly, I say to you, whoever does not receive the kingdom of God as a little child will by no means enter it." 16 And He took them up in His arms, put His hands on them, and blessed them.

Lk 1:46-49 And Mary said: "My soul magnifies the Lord, 47 and my spirit has rejoiced in God my Savior. 48 for He has regarded the lowly state of His maidservant; For behold, henceforth all generations will call me blessed. 49 For He who is mighty has done great things for me, and holy is His name.

Good Health

3 Jn 1:2, "Beloved, I pray that in all respects you may prosper and be in good health, just as your soul prospers." (NASB)

PRAYERS

Prayer shows loving concern and is a means of bringing comfort, spiritual assurance, confidence in decision making, and peace in the midst of the patient's health crises. Prayer creates an atmosphere in which the presence of God is felt and where the Holy Spirit is invited to comfort, minister, and guide. If applied sensitively and timely it can also enhance the relationship between the patient and the intercessor. Be sure and ask the patient what they would like you to include in the prayer. Pray scripture, there is power in the Word!

When praying do not project as a "faith healer". Ultimately we must accept that God has a plan and purpose for each life. While death is an interruption of God's perfect plan, that we were to live forever, it is a reality of the consequences of sin and our life on this earth. In Isaiah 57:1-2 we are instructed that, "The righteous perish and no one ponders it in his heart; devout men are taken away, and no one understands that the righteous are taken away to be spared from evil. Those who walk uprightly enter into peace; and they find rest as they lie in death." We do not know when it is the end of one's time on this earth. We can pray our heart, claim God's promises, and ask for God's will that His destiny for the patient be fulfilled. In some cases it is okay if the patient chooses death. Be sensitive to the situation and to God's voice.

Of Commitment

If the person is accepting Jesus as their Lord and Savior have them repeat this prayer after you.

Dear Heavenly Father, I believe that Jesus Christ is Your only begotten Son. I believe that He became a man and died on the cross, to pay the penalty for my sins that were separating me from You. I believe that he was buried and rose from the dead physically, to give me new life.

Lord Jesus, I ask You to forgive my sins. I receive You as my Lord and Savior. I ask You to come into my heart. I believe that You have forgiven my sins and have come into my heart. I thank You for Your promise of eternal life given in Your Word. John 3:36 says that, "He who believes in the Son has everlasting life; and he who does not believe the Son shall not see life, but the wrath of God abides on him." And in 2 Corinthians 5:1 "Therefore, if anyone is in Christ, he is a new creation; old things have passed away; behold, all things have become new.

Thank You for Your sacrifice and victory. Thank You for Your love. Thank You that this is a time of new beginnings. I choose You and new life. In Jesus name, Amen

Grieving

"O Holy One, Our Father and Our God, teach us how to grieve. Give us the courage to acknowledge our pain, to hold it awhile and then to set it free. Give us the strength to choose to move beyond what has altered our life forever, to find a new normal; a new life where precious memories bring gladness. Help us to honor new beginnings by building upon our memories a life of joy and hope. We will be gentle with ourselves and with each other during this process and take time to grieve and heal. Thank you for carrying us through this journey. In Jesus name, Amen." (by Karen Johnston)

The Lord's Prayer

"Our Father which art in heaven, Hallowed be Thy name. Thy kingdom come. Thy will be done in earth, as it is in heaven. Give us this day our daily bread. And forgive us our debts(trespasses) as we forgive our debtors (those who trespass against us). And lead us not into temptation, but deliver us from evil: For Thine is the kingdom, and the power, and the glory, forever. Amen" (Matthew 6:9-13)

CPSIA information can be obtained at www.ICGtesting.com
Printed in the USA
BVOW011629290313

316842BV00003B/7/P

9 781626 520691